Church End
ary
3800
KT-418-807

THE
MIND
MEDIC

30131 05718199 9

LONDON BOROUGH OF BARNET

DR SARAH VOHRA

THE
MIND
MEDIC

Your 5 Senses Guide to Leading
a Calmer, Happier Life

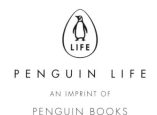

PENGUIN LIFE

AN IMPRINT OF

PENGUIN BOOKS

PENGUIN LIFE

UK | USA | Canada | Ireland | Australia
India | New Zealand | South Africa

Penguin Life is part of the Penguin Random House group of companies
whose addresses can be found at global.penguinrandomhouse.com.

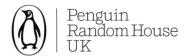

First published 2020
001

Copyright © Dr Sarah Vohra, 2020

The moral right of the author has been asserted

Designed by Hampton
Colour reproduction by Rhapsody Ltd
Printed and bound in Germany by Firmengruppe APPL, Aprinta Druck GmbH

A CIP catalogue record for this book is available from the British Library

ISBN: 978–0–241–42189–5

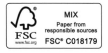

Penguin Random House is committed to a sustainable future for our
business, our readers and our planet. This book is made from Forest
Stewardship Council® certified paper.

For Amelie and Ravi

CONTENTS

Introduction **8**

The 5 senses 10

Chapter 1: SEE **15**

Screen use 16

Social media 24

Body image 31

Change your outlook 43

Choosing the people you see 51

Chapter 2: HEAR **61**

Hear yourself 62

Just say 'no' 78

Mark of approval 86

Start to hear compliments 93

Taking criticism on the chin 104

Chapter 3: SMELL **110**

Breathe in: mindfulness and meditation 111

The smell of the great outdoors 113

Smelling the bullshit 120

Sweet smell of success 126

Scents, sleep and all things self-care 137

Chapter 4: FEEL   146

Time to worry 147

Perfectly imperfect 154

Feel confident in your own skin 164

Lightening the load when feeling under pressure ... 171

Stop feeling like an impostor 177

Chapter 5: TASTE   182

Food glorious food 183

Keeping it regular 191

Throwing out the rule book 195

The drug and supplement trap 216

Revenge tastes so sweet 230

Chapter 6: The 5 Senses Plan: Bringing It All Together   239

Epilogue: Let Your Senses Be Your Guide   250

References   252

Acknowledgements   255

INTRODUCTION

The lives we lead every day have become more demanding. We are constantly connected in a way that we weren't 10 or 20 years ago. We barely have a minute to breathe and unwind from the stresses of the day before we find ourselves snoozing our morning alarm, ready to jump back on the hamster wheel and do it all over again.

Sound familiar?

All these demands on our time and energy can impact our mental health. Dressed up in various guises, whether it's 'wellness', 'wellbeing' or 'self-care', the advice available to us is vast and can feel incredibly overwhelming. What is *actually* going to make a difference to our mental wellbeing?

The advice that we are given routinely is simply to 'talk more'. And while this is important, for many it isn't enough simply to share their emotional struggles with somebody else. Yes, it gets *it* out into the open and it can be encouraging to hear that someone understands or has experienced a similar hardship, but all too often what are missing are simple tools or strategies that you can use to get yourself out of that lull and optimize how you feel. Even if someone does offer you strategies that have worked for them, there is no guarantee that they will work for you.

We are all hardwired differently. Life experiences and events can affect us all in different ways. Why is it that some of us naturally shine on stage whereas the rest of us come out in hives at the prospect of a work presentation? Why is it that some of us can escape a car crash relatively unscathed (both mentally and physically) while others vow never to get behind the wheel again? We all have different tools available to us, from the external help and support we get from our relationships and physical environment to our own internal coping mechanisms and behaviours that we can draw upon to help us to navigate our way through life.

As a consultant psychiatrist, I have worked with thousands of patients to help them overcome a whole host of mental health difficulties, from relationship break-ups and stresses at work to the more serious clinical disorders such as depression and anxiety, where some individuals are rendered housebound and may even contemplate not wanting to be alive any more. While with the latter patients we may start them on medication (at least for the short term) to help manage their symptoms, the core of their treatment and recovery, the 'getting them back to fighting fit', is in helping them better understand their difficulties and empowering them to learn and develop practical tools to best manage these.

The two most common questions I get asked by my patients in clinic are how can I keep myself 'mentally healthy', and how do I pick myself up if and when I do hit a rocky patch? I tell them that half the battle is in them being able to recognize early on when things aren't quite right (these signs can look and feel very different for each of us), and the other half is in learning to develop a toolbox of tried-and-tested methods, individual to them, which can be called upon at any given moment to help. It has been ingrained in us from day dot that eating well and exercising regularly is a sure-fire way of ensuring our physical health is in tip-top condition. We also know that when we have had a health scare, the food we eat and how much we move play a pivotal role in our recovery. But do we know what we ought to be doing to make ourselves more mentally healthy? And would we have the faintest idea of how to pull ourselves out of a rocky patch?

The practical tips and tools I share in this book are ones I use routinely with the patients I work with. The simple 5-step method will, I hope, empower you also to develop a personalized toolkit to survive the emotional twists and turns that this modern world can bring. I want to help you reclaim your mental wellbeing and be the happiest, healthiest version of yourself.

I wish you the best of luck on your journey.

Sarah x

THE 5 SENSES

The 5 senses plan is a simple method to help you pinpoint your life stresses, develop simple solutions to manage them and reclaim your inner calm.

You experience the world through your senses: your sight, hearing, smell, sense of touch (feel) and taste. Your sensory organs – eyes, ears, nose, skin and mouth – help you to perceive, interact with and explore your environment. Linked to your brain via your nervous system, your 5 senses help you to determine what you think about a given experience, how you feel about it (the good and the bad) and, crucially, how you then go on to act.

There may be times when you struggle to put your finger on what it is about a particular day or interaction that means your mood takes a turn for the worse. What I teach my patients to do is think about whether there is anything they may have **seen, heard, smelled, felt** or **tasted** (not necessarily all at once) that could possibly provide an explanation.

It may be that you have *seen* something negative on social media (SEE) or spent the afternoon with an overly critical boss (HEAR). Maybe you overlooked your usual daily breathwork (SMELL) or woke up feeling less than perfect (FEEL). Perhaps it is only mid-morning but you're on to your second double espresso to get you through a particularly busy work shift (TASTE). I encourage my patients to perform this simple exercise, which helps them to piece together the jigsaw of the day and identify possible stresses.

Throughout this book, I invite you to think about your life experiences in this way, as a culmination of your senses.

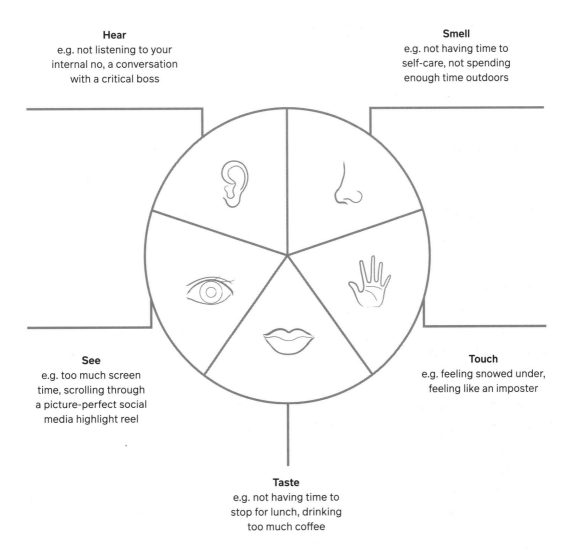

Hear
e.g. not listening to your internal no, a conversation with a critical boss

Smell
e.g. not having time to self-care, not spending enough time outdoors

See
e.g. too much screen time, scrolling through a picture-perfect social media highlight reel

Touch
e.g. feeling snowed under, feeling like an imposter

Taste
e.g. not having time to stop for lunch, drinking too much coffee

'Ask yourself' and '5 sense challenge' sections feature throughout the book.

Ask yourself gives you a space to reflect on your own experiences and will help you work out whether the sense being described is a difficulty for you at the moment. If so, it encourages you to think about what changes you might like to make and what obstacles might be getting in your way.

The **5 sense challenge** gives you practical solutions to overcome these obstacles.

The wellbeing thermometer

The wellbeing thermometer is a tool I regularly use in clinic. You may well find yourself experiencing a range of different emotions throughout the day; in much the same way that your body temperature can change over a 24-hour period, your *wellbeing* can also experience similar spikes and drops in temperature.

The wellbeing thermometer icon will appear throughout the book. Where you see it, I want you to draw a horizontal arrow pointing at the level that best corresponds to how you feel.

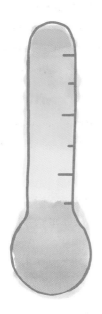

Red: Mostly negative feelings that make life experiences unbearable, e.g. not attending social events or going to work.

Orange: Negative feelings that lead you to contemplate opting out of life experiences – and sometimes to turn them down – e.g. occasionally cancelling social events or pulling a sickie.

Yellow: Feelings that might make you uncomfortable but do not interfere too much with life experiences.

Green: Generally positive feelings – if you do experience any negative feelings, these are dealt with easily and do not affect life experiences.

Blue: Mostly positive feelings that do not affect life experiences.

When you anticipate a heatwave, you plan ahead. You may pack some sun cream or a pair of sunglasses. The point being that you equip yourself with the tools you need that will make you feel comfortable and any change in temperature more bearable.

While you may not be able to avoid the reds and oranges – stresses at work, for instance, are inevitable – you can adapt how you respond to them, reduce the stress they cause you and cool your wellbeing temperature.

By using the wellbeing thermometer to record your *temperature* you can start to identify which senses are causing you the most stress and therefore may be the most important to work on.

You may choose to overlook areas where your wellbeing temperature is already blue and jump ahead to those where you are regularly scoring reds and oranges. That is absolutely fine. Some sections or even senses in the book may not be areas of difficulty for you at the moment. You may have experienced them in the past and come through the other side, or they may be something you will come to experience in the future. If that's the case, you can dip in to the relevant sense chapter as and when you need to and adapt your plan accordingly.

This book is not about being prescriptive or needing to follow each suggestion to the letter, but rather ensuring that you develop a plan that is individual to you and your difficulties right now.

The final chapter, Chapter 6, will guide you in developing your personalized 5 senses plan: a 10-week programme to help you reclaim your mental wellbeing and be the happiest, healthiest version of yourself.

The 5 senses overview

See	Hear	Smell	Feel	Taste
Screen use	Hear yourself	Breathe in: mindfulness and meditation	Time to worry	Food glorious food
Social media	Just say 'no'	The smell of the great outdoors	Perfectly imperfect	Keeping it regular
Body image	Mark of approval	Smelling the bullshit	Feel confident in your own skin	Throwing out the rule book
Change your outlook	Start to hear compliments	Sweet smell of success	Lightening the load when feeling under pressure	The drug and supplement trap
Choosing the people you see	Taking criticism on the chin	Scents, sleep and all things self-care	Stop feeling like an impostor	Revenge tastes so sweet

Chapter 1
SEE

Screen use

I have no doubt that screen use has some role to play in the stresses of our everyday lives. Certainly with some of the patients I see, there is always some means of tracing their symptoms back to the use, or rather over-use, of a screen, from spending too much time on devices before bed to prioritizing online 'friendships' over in-real-life (IRL) or face-to-face connections. It might be that they blur the boundaries between work and rest by actioning an email late at night, or find themselves down a social media rabbit-hole of comparison. Such behaviours stand to negatively impact their mood, confidence, anxiety levels and sleep.

While we are far from being able to determine a cause and effect, i.e. that screen use causes negative mental wellbeing, the studies that do exist certainly suggest that increased screen use can be of detriment. To be clear, the literature available tends to focus very much on screen use *in general* rather than differentiating the different types of screen use, and where studies do exist that capture the latter, these appear to be limited to television, use of phone for texting and computer use. And even then, it is difficult to tease out whether it is screen use per se that is the problem or the purpose for which it is being used.

Several studies have shown that increased levels of screen time (7 hours or more per day) are associated with an increased risk of depression, with some even suggesting screen use as a risk factor for anxiety, particularly in children and adolescents. This appears to be especially problematic when coupled with less physical activity. It has also been shown to impact attention levels. There has even been some evidence that suggests that combined high use of computers (more than 4 hours per day) and phones is associated with prolonged stress and depression, particularly in women.

We know that using blue light emitting diode (LED) devices such as smartphones, laptops and tablets at night can impact our natural sleep rhythm, reducing the quality of our sleep, and can even go on to impact our mood, concentration and energy levels the following day. Certainly the evidence supports the association between high screen time and sleep disturbance. The blue LED light blocks the release of a hormone called melatonin by almost 25%. Melatonin release is crucial in triggering the pathways for onset of sleep.

While it is far from realistic to introduce a blanket ban on our devices or to start recommending optimal 'doses' of screen time, we can learn to set sensible limits on our usage, particularly where we notice them negatively impacting our mental wellbeing.

Setting limits

From doing our online food shop to paying for a coffee; scheduling diary appointments to taking notes during a lecture or meeting; searching for recipe inspiration to unwinding with a book before bed, screens are everywhere. While all these advances help us lead more efficient lives (a plus for our mental wellbeing), how do we protect ourselves from becoming too dependent on them, using them as a means to procrastinate and potentially lose touch with the 'real' world around us (a minus for our mental wellbeing)? How can we strike a happy medium that means our screen use doesn't start to negatively impact our mood, disrupt our sleep or make us feel anxious?

It's safe to say that screens are here to stay, so we need to learn to foster healthier relationships with them. One of the most impactful ways of achieving a healthy balance is to limit the amount of time we spend staring at them. We can now track and limit our screen time within our devices. If this is something you do, what *actually* happens when you hit your limit? I know from personal experience that the temptation to override is great and all too easy. You might choose to make an exception '*just this once*' for something that you '*have to post*' or for an email that you '*have to send*', but before you know it you are overriding the limit daily and may even be bold enough to remove the limits set altogether.

So, what is causing you to spend so much time on your devices? Can you justify all your phone use, for instance, as being 'absolutely essential'?

THE 5 SENSE CHALLENGE:
log in

To get a better understanding of your personal use, I like to divide screen use into three distinct categories: the Not Entirely Necessary, the Non-negotiable and the Like to Do.

The **Not Entirely Necessary** (NEN) are the times where you pick up your phone, push back the screen of your laptop or turn on your tablet through sheer habit. You are not quite sure why you have unlocked your phone or how you got to scrolling your social media feed, but you are there now. Before long you have squandered minutes, if not hours, on mindless consumption.

The **Non-negotiable** (NN) are the times you use your screens because you have a **clear purpose**, at a particular time or to maintain **positive** connections with others. The emails that need sending; the phone calls or texting for work, or to catch up with family or friends. Online banking, filling in a tax return, pulling up a recipe to follow for dinner or doing that online shop.

The **Like to Do** (LTD) are the things that you enjoy doing but that are **not** *absolutely* **essential**. This could include binge-watching the latest box set, listening to a podcast or getting lost in a Pinterest mood board. LTDs don't have to be done at a specific time, nor do they have any time constraints set upon them in the way that NNs do. While the LTDs are arguably just as important as the NNs by giving you the opportunity to unwind and relax, you need to be careful that they don't start to negatively impact your mental wellbeing. For instance, binge-watching box sets late at night may impact your sleep and affect your mood, energy and concentration levels the following day. Or casually scrolling a social media highlights reel may see your body image insecurities triggered by *that* one image.

Using the screen log opposite, tally up **every** time you use a screen (phone, laptop, computer, tablet, e-reader or TV). It may be helpful to compare different days of the week. For instance, a working versus non-working day, where your screen use may vary.

Before recording your screen use, think about how this particular activity has made you feel.

A NEN morning scroll sees you procrastinating from an important project (**RED**), feeling stressed responding to a NN work email mid-afternoon (**ORANGE**), or feeling calm unwinding with a LTD podcast in the evening (**BLUE**). Use a corresponding coloured pencil to tally your screen use in the relevant time slot.

Example of screen log:

	Morning	Afternoon	Evening	Total	Notes
NEN	| | | |	| | |	| | | |		
NN	| | |	| | | |	| | |		
LTD	| |		| | | |		

Daily screen logs:

MON	Morning	Afternoon	Evening	Total	Notes
NEN					
NN					
LTD					

TUE	Morning	Afternoon	Evening	Total	Notes
NEN					
NN					
LTD					

WED	Morning	Afternoon	Evening	Total	Notes
NEN					
NN					
LTD					

THR	Morning	Afternoon	Evening	Total	Notes
NEN					
NN					
LTD					

FRI	Morning	Afternoon	Evening	Total	Notes
NEN					
NN					
LTD					

SAT	Morning	Afternoon	Evening	Total	Notes
NEN					
NN					
LTD					

SUN	Morning	Afternoon	Evening	Total	Notes
NEN					
NN					
LTD					

At the start of the day, write down the NNs, the tasks you absolutely *have* to do. Ask yourself whether these have to be completed today, or can they be spread out throughout the week?

Think about the LTDs for that day. Schedule these in and around your NNs.

Next set aside a window each day of 30 minutes to an hour for some mindless scrolling, the NENs.

Throughout the day, each time you reach for your screen and find yourself drawn into a NEN, remind yourself of your allocated window. Stop the scroll in its tracks and return to the activity you are doing with the knowledge that you have permission to do this later.

Ask yourself

When do you use your screen? Morning, afternoon or evening?

....

What is your overall wellbeing temperature? What colour stands out from your screen log?

....

Do the NENs, the NNs or the LTDs occupy most of your screen time?

....

Does a certain type of screen use (NEN, NN or LTD) see your wellbeing temperature rise more than others?

....

Start the day right

For many of us, the need to be connected starts the moment we wake up, when we turn off our phone alarm. However, replacing our regular alarm clock with our phone can see us enticed by what else it has to offer. Typically what follows is the inevitable overnight notifications check. Any text messages? Missed phone calls? How about emails? You might then scroll through your various social media accounts to catch up on what your friends, family members, celebrities or favourite influencers have been up to – all of this before you have even got yourself out of bed.

How does your morning routine make you feel?

Depending on what you look at, checking your screen can dictate how you feel and behave in the morning, whether it is panicking over that work email you are convinced needs actioning before you even step foot in the shower, or feeling guilty over your snoozed alarm when faced with someone else's post-gym selfie. It is time to reclaim your morning routine.

THE 5 SENSE CHALLENGE:
reclaim your morning

Charge your phone out of the bedroom. If it must be in there, put it out of arm's reach so you have to physically get out of bed to retrieve it.

Invest in a regular alarm clock. Avoid relying on your phone as your wake-up call. Get out of the habit of using your phone as a 'catch all' for all your daily tasks, particularly where there are reasonable alternatives.

Avoid looking at your phone during the first hour of waking. Place your phone and devices on airplane mode to enable you to carry out your morning routine interruption-free, rather than allowing incoming notifications to set your morning pace.

Notes

....

....

....

....

....

....

Social media

Advances in social media mean that we are more connected than ever before. These platforms allow us to express ourselves and to create and maintain meaningful connections with others. And while I don't dispute these benefits, our need to be constantly switched on, always available and at the beck and call of others and with a plethora of images and words at our fingertips, it can be all too easy to feel overwhelmed and fall foul of the downsides of social media. The Royal Society for Public Health has shown that social media can impact our sleep, worsen anxiety and depression, instil worries about body image and heighten our fear of missing out. Certainly this is the picture that is reflected in my clinic room.

While we are not yet able to establish a cause and effect, i.e. that social media *causes* negative mental wellbeing, this double-edged sword has seen some studies alluding to the idea that it is dose-dependent, i.e. the longer you spend on social media the more harmful it can be.

In 2018, the *Economist* shed light on the link between the heavy use of social media and mental illness in an article that extrapolated data from Moment, an activity-tracking app. Each week, Moment routinely surveys its 1 million users and evaluates their use of social networking sites including Facebook, Instagram, Snapchat and Twitter and how happy they are about said use. It found that 63% of Instagram users report being miserable, which is a higher share than for any other social networking site (SNS), with users typically spending an hour per day on the app; conversely, the 37% who reported feeling content spent only half as long. This observation certainly supports the idea that the length of time spent on social media is important.

The literature also highlights that the highly curated nature of social media content means that we are seeing more of the upward social comparisons where we compare ourselves to others who we perceive to 'have it all' or who are in some way superior to us; presenting your 'best self' is often the premise of most SNS. It is these upward comparisons that are thought to be detrimental to our mental wellbeing.

The smoke and mirror effect

Our online presence has hyped up social comparisons. You now have the ability to compare yourself to anyone, at any time, from celebrities halfway across the world, to your friends and peers. And the comparisons start from the moment you get up right through to the moment you go to sleep; from beautifully arranged breakfast bowls to #selfcare evening routines, everything is fair game.

We know deep down that social media is just a highlights reel. How many of us share an image of ourselves on an 'off day'? You also don't see the 99 photos that came before the one that made the cut. You don't see the time sacrificed (time with a partner, time that could otherwise be spent eating), the perfect lighting and the makeup that come together in synchrony to get that 'perfect shot'.

On a recent holiday with my husband and daughter I came face to face with the embodiment of the social media 'smoke and mirrors effect'. Sitting at the breakfast buffet I couldn't help but notice a couple to our left; neither would have looked out of place on the cover of a health and fitness magazine. Their table was adorned with buffet offerings, from coffee, green juices, a platter of fruits and scrambled eggs to towering pancakes and waffles. Several photos, a series of Instagram stories to capture their epic spread and barely a swig of coffee between them later, they made a swift exit, leaving the food on the table untouched.

You may ask yourself, what's the harm? On the one hand, some of their followers may be inspired and motivated by their content – '*They are eating all this great food and look how [insert desirable body aesthetic here] they are*' – but on the other hand there may be those for whom it fuels feelings of inadequacy – '*I wish I had more self-control on holiday*' or '*Why can't I eat all that food and look like them?*'

The truth of the matter is **there is no truth**, and if you feel the pressure of comparison you are ultimately basing your worth on a) someone you more than likely have never met, and b) someone who is only showing you a glimpse of the full story.

So what's the solution? How do you avoid being drawn into the vortex of social media comparison?

THE 5 SENSE CHALLENGE:
curate your
social media feed

While it may feel at times that you are fighting a losing battle with constantly changing algorithms, it is important to remember that **you** are in control of your own social media feeds. That colourful breakfast that you see first thing in the morning, those perfectly carved abs and that young man or woman who just seems to '*have it all*' – you are *choosing* to follow them. You have consciously 'followed them', perhaps blinded by number of followers, status, the circles they move in or that alluring blue tick. You convince yourself that following them will inspire or motivate you. You convince yourself that you *need* to make a change and to be *more like them in order to achieve happiness, success and even love*. But their daily posts only serve to remind you that you are '*not quite there yet*', and can mean your often flailing self-esteem spirals down even further.

It. Never. Ends.

Unless, of course, you brave the 'unfollow'.

Sounds simple, right? But this decision can see us deliberating, but ultimately concluding that it is safer to continue to follow regardless of the impact that it may be having on our mental wellbeing.

Ask yourself, is this content relevant to me **right now**?
Does it make me feel good and/or positive?
If the answer is NO to both, brave an **unfollow**.

For many the 'unfollow' is a silent sin. Something to be avoided at all costs, for fear of bumping into the unfollowed or the embarrassment of re-following. A compromise, if the unfollow feels too bold a move, could be to mute the account. Although you continue to 'follow' them, their content will no longer pop up on your feed. This gives you the option to un-mute them at a later date.

Social media: how do you use it?

While we have focused on the accounts you follow, it is equally important to shed the spotlight on your own role as an 'influencer'. And you *are* an influencer – you don't have to have tens of thousands of followers to be of '*influence*'. Any content you put out into the public domain is a means of influencing others in some shape or form. Why do you upload that family photo or holiday snap to Facebook or Instagram, share that selfie via Snapchat or get enraged with a Twitter debate?

Maybe you have uploaded a sunny holiday snap to your socials when you know full well it is nothing but rain and showers back home. You can usually predict the response doing so will get. Yet every like and envious comment from family and friends reinforces '*how lucky you are*'.

Perhaps you have embarked on a health and fitness journey and have made a remarkable transformation. Feeling bold, you upload a selfie on to your socials. Your journey may spark questions on how you did it and nudge family and friends to embark on a transformation of their own. Every like and every positive comment validates the wonderful transformation you have undergone and boosts your self-esteem.

The growth of social media has broadened our influence. You now have the ability to influence individuals who more often than not you have never met. You may no longer seek validation from a family member, close friend or work colleague but you yearn for that hypothetical nod from complete strangers through follows, likes and positive comments.

The problem? By placing expectation on others to *approve* your actions, you unknowingly give them permission to decide how you feel about yourself, your ability and your choices: your **self-esteem**. When we seek external validation, our decision to celebrate or feel confident about our choices becomes dependent on someone else's measure of success. Why should a caption you are proud of, or an outfit you like and feel confident in, suddenly leave you plagued with self-doubt because it has been 'proved otherwise' by others?

Ask yourself

To help you work out whether your social media use is problematic, ask yourself the following questions.

Are your notifications for social media accounts permanently on?

....

Do you find yourself going on to your social media account every time you receive a notification informing you of a new follower, a like or a new comment?

....

Do you find that you are spending minutes to hours planning what to post, at the expense of other activities in your day?

....

Do you find that after you post something you are religiously checking and refreshing the page to check the level of engagement?

....

Does your mood get affected if your post does not get the level of engagement you anticipate?

....

Have you ever deleted a post because of the poor level of engagement it has received, even if you wholeheartedly believed in its message?

....

Do you know the number of followers you have right down to the last individual?

....

Do you keep track of when someone has unfollowed you? Do you actively engage that individual in discussion, asking why they have unfollowed you?

....

Do you find yourself drawing comparisons to others online?

....

If five or more of the questions above ring true for you, it may indicate that your social media use is becoming a problem and it is probably worth considering how you tailor your use, particularly if it is having a negative impact on your mental wellbeing.

THE 5 SENSE CHALLENGE:
tailoring your social media use

Here are my top tips for reducing your wellbeing temperature and improving your relationship with social media.

Switch off all push notifications across all your social media channels. Every buzz, beep or screen banner informing you of a new like, comment or follower can mean you never truly escape its grips, being connected or the need to be externally validated. It may serve as a reminder, a way of pulling you back in to check that comment or who that new follower is, and can make sticking to the boundaries you set yourself all the more difficult.

Be authentic. Post what you wish to post and not what you feel you *ought* to be posting.

Ask yourself, why? Why am I posting this particular content at this moment in time? Why can't it wait until later, if at all? If there is no clear purpose, then do not post it.

Quit the refresh. When you do post, enter a contract with yourself that you will not monitor its engagement. If you have decided that you are choosing to post for **you**, then it is important to be unapologetic about that and not seek validation based on the level of engagement you receive. I have worked with patients who constantly refresh their social media pages after uploading a post or photo, and will go on to actively remove the post when it doesn't get enough likes or when they receive a negative comment.

Of course, you may be someone who positively thrives on the engagement you get or who actively encourages debate even from those who are saying less than favourable things, in which case refreshing may not negatively impact your mental wellbeing and may be just a means of keeping track of threads, particularly with fast-paced SNS such as Twitter.

Stop stalking your followers. If you lose followers, that is not a reflection on you as an individual. For whatever reason your content isn't serving them right now, that's OK. They may come back to you. They may not. Take their lead and let it motivate you to spring-clean the accounts you follow, rather than let it dishearten you.

Body image

Over a third of UK adults have felt anxious or depressed about their body image. I know from personal experience how detrimental thinking and feeling negatively about your body can be. As a teen, I didn't like how I looked. I struggled with severe acne and was deemed by others to be 'overweight'. I tormented myself, drawing comparisons with friends, random passers-by and the 'perfect bodies' that adorned the weekly glossies. It almost certainly affected what ought to have been simple decisions at my age – what I ate, what I wore and whether I went out or not. I felt I ought to eat less, cover up and steer clear of socials. It was only after becoming a mum that I realized the way I thought and felt about my body – my body image – was really becoming quite detrimental. I had started to measure my success not on what goals I had achieved in life but on whether I fitted society's aesthetic ideal while achieving them. School proms, university nights out, graduations, holidays and the pre-wedding excitement – occasions I won't get back and all marred by needing to look a certain way; a way predetermined by other people, not myself. I realized that I didn't want that for my daughter growing up. I didn't want her to determine her worth by how she looked, but by what she could do. For the last five years, I have changed the language I use when talking about my body. I do not talk negatively about my body outwardly to my husband or in front of her. I look in the mirror each morning and while I may not always like what I see, I am at peace with it. I accept my body flaws and view these differences as what sets me apart from other people. I remind myself of what my body can do and where it has got me.

2,500 women were surveyed as part of *Women's Health UK* Project Body Love 2019 campaign. Out of these 2,500, only 6% agreed with the statement 'I love my body.' If this rings true for you, feeling dissatisfied with your body image might affect your self-confidence and your interaction with others; you may be more likely to steer clear of social gatherings or feel incredibly uncomfortable and self-conscious attending them. It can lower your mood, increase anxiety and see you harbour unhealthy relationships with food. Worryingly, 1 in 8 UK adults have even experienced suicidal thoughts because of a negative body image.

Conversely, body image satisfaction is associated with better overall wellbeing and less unhealthy dieting behaviour. Your body image can be influenced by a number of factors including your friendships and relationships, how those around you feel and speak about their bodies as well as pressure from the media or social media pushing the 'ideal'. Of those surveyed by the Mental Health Foundation and YouGov, 20% cite images on social media as a factor for body dissatisfaction. The Dove Global Beauty and Confidence Report (Unilever 2017) found that 60% of females believe that social media pressures them to look a certain way, with 70% believing media and advertising set an unrealistic standard of beauty.

The Ideal

Society's expectations of 'the ideal' body shape are constantly changing, from 'heroin-chic' to 'strong is the new skinny' this decade. Often the ideal body shape of the moment is pushed forward and heavily marketed by the health, beauty, fashion and diet industries, ready to prey on our vulnerabilities. By defining the ideal, these multi-million-pound industries are creating a problem we may never have thought existed, and jump in to offer us the often costly 'solutions'.

Time for some honesty. When you look in the mirror, what is the first thing that you **think** about or comment on?

*How do you **feel** when you look in the mirror? Record your temperature using the wellbeing thermometer.*

How does the way you think and feel about your body affect how you then go on to **act**?

That initial mirror check in the morning can hold so much power over you. If you look in the mirror and like what you see, you carry yourself with more confidence and feel better prepared to tackle the day ahead.

However, if you don't like what's staring back at you, you might choose to 'cover up' or to turn down an invite for fear of how you look and may be viewed by others. It might influence how you behave in your friendships and relationships. It might even distract you from what you are doing at work.

If you struggle with your body image, you can stop living in the moment and pass on opportunities that come your way. You might even believe, as certainly some of the patients I see have, that happiness, success or love will only come to you *when* you reach a certain size or weight.

I know when I scroll through social media or flick through a magazine it is hard not to get drawn into marketing ploys that sell you an ideal of how you *should* look, and it is only natural that they lead you to draw comparisons and affect the confidence you have in your own skin. If you regularly struggle with poor body image, thinking about your body and your perceived flaws can be exhausting and all-consuming.

Ask yourself

What does the perfect body look like to you?

....

....

....

What do you think that this body would bring you?

....

....

....

Where do you think these ideas have come from?

....

....

....

Looking back at your early years, what do you think shaped your relationship with your body?

....

....

....

How did you feel about your body growing up?

....

....

....

Were comments frequently made about your body by others?

....

....

....

How did those around you – parents, family and friends – talk about their own bodies?

....

....

....

Have your ideas about the 'perfect body' been shaped by what you have seen in the media or on social media?

....

....

....

THE 5 SENSE CHALLENGE:
mirror mirror

Learn to practise mind and body gratitude **daily**. Each morning, when you look in the mirror, really take note of what you see and challenge those immediate negative thoughts that come to the forefront. For each negative thought you might have about yourself, challenge yourself to match it with a positive.

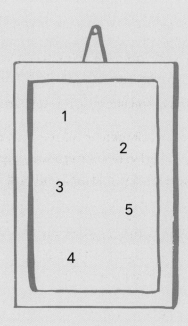

Look at yourself as a whole (inside and out) and stop focusing on the aesthetic only. Challenge yourself to come up with 5 things that you like about yourself.

1. ....

2. ....

3. ....

4. ....

5. ....

To help you out, you might like to:

- Think about what your body can **do**. What will it help you accomplish that day – both physically and mentally?
- What positive qualities and personality traits do you possess?

Put this list somewhere you can easily see (on your mirror) or refer to (notes section on your phone). The next time you find yourself negatively body-talking, stop the thought in its tracks, pull out your list, remind yourself of, and positively affirm, what your body *can* do.

Early studies have shown that practising self-affirmation enables you to view yourself more positively, to be more satisfied with your body self-image and to be less likely to use body weight and shape as a means of evaluating yourself.

Meet Ros:

Ros is 27 and has had a poor relationship with her body over the years. She has yo-yo dieted for most of her teens and twenties. She has starved herself, tried the latest fad shake or diet pills. She has bought clothes in smaller sizes in a bid to 'slim down into them'. The clothes she does wear are uncomfortable and serve as a reminder that she needs to slim down. She refuses to buy the next size up. She steps on the scale each morning and berates herself when she has not lost any weight or, worse still, if she has gained. If it is the latter, then she spends the day restricting only to cave at the eleventh hour and to binge her way through the evening. If she steps on the scales and it is a number that she likes, she feels lighter mentally – happier and more confident. Ros tracks what she eats – a calorie over and she criticizes herself over her lack of control – and she believes that she is and will remain fat.

Ros told me that her ideals around body types are based on what she sees on social media and in glossy magazines. She finds the same aesthetic everywhere she turns, and believes this is genuinely how she needs to look to be desirable or successful. She trusts that she will be happier once she gets down to that certain size or weight.

I wondered why Ros didn't feel or believe that these things could come now, at the size that she is currently. There seemed to be a lot of 'ifs' and 'whens'. Ros accepted that she was putting a lot of things on hold until she had lost the weight, from buying new clothes, to signing up to a dating app, to going for a promotion at work.

Ros accepted that she did not believe she was worthy of happiness or success unless she fitted society's unrealistic expectations. She sought approval for how she looked from those around her ('in real life' and online) and from the number on the scales or inside a clothing label. This meant that when things were going well (she received a compliment, the number on the scale was desirable or she got down to a particular dress size) she was 'being good' or had 'self-control', but when faced with no compliments, a stubborn scale and struggling to squeeze herself into a smaller dress size, she perceived herself as being 'bad' or 'lacking willpower or self-control'. These markers served as her moral compass.

Ros forfeited her self-esteem to other people and objects to determine. This meant that Ros was not able to develop it for herself. Even if Ros woke up feeling confident and optimistic about the day ahead, this could very quickly unravel as soon as she stepped foot on the scales, whose number would determine that 'she shouldn't feel confident' and her day would be anything but optimistic.

*Ros recognized that in order to become more accepting (and hopefully in time, confident) of the body she is in **now**, she had to let go of those external measures (the need for approval from others, the scales, the 'ideal' dress size) that could very quickly derail any progress she made with this.*

Ros was gradually able to let go of these external measures and weaken the hold they had over her. She binned the scales and, while she found the 'unknown of her weight' unnerving to begin with, she started to feel more liberated over the fact that her mood for the day suddenly wasn't determined or dependent on a number. She felt more in control than she had ever felt.

Similarly, she rediscovered her love for shopping and bought herself clothes that fitted her body right now. She realized how much importance she had placed on numbers and how meaningless they were in the grand scheme of what else she had to offer. She realized that she didn't view her close friends and family as a number. She measured these relationships and friendships on how they made her feel and the qualities each individual bears, and it was likely that they similarly wouldn't view her as such, a number.

Liberating herself from these external measures meant that Ros was able to start working on building her self-esteem back up without the threat of it being derailed by a size or number.

THE 5 SENSE CHALLENGE:
the 7-day ditch

I have listed the most common objects that patients I see use to define how they think, feel and behave. Do any of these sound familiar to you?

For each of the below, record your wellbeing temperature.

- Subscribed emails
- Social media
- Clothes labels
- Fitness watch, pedometer or activity tracker
- Food tracking app
- Kitchen scales or measuring utensils
- Bathroom scales

Over the next 7 days, challenge yourself to ditch or unsubscribe from one troublesome object at a time; from the least feared (blue) to the most feared (red). Your 7-day ditch may look a little something like this:

Monday
Unsubscribe from any spam emails that land in your inbox promising you the latest miracle diet cure or coaxing you into the latest health and fitness plan.

Tuesday
Curate your social media feed and unfollow or mute those accounts that routinely make you feel inadequate about your body.

Wednesday
Have a wardrobe clear-out and get rid of all the clothes that don't fit and that you have promised yourself you will '*squeeze into one day*'.

Thursday
If you have one, rethink the purpose of your fitness watch or pedometer. If it is solely there as a means of holding you accountable for what you eat and how much you move, then it is time to get rid.

Friday
If you have one, delete your food tracking app from your phone and any other devices.

Saturday
Get rid of the kitchen scales if you are using them as a means of controlling your portion size for every meal or snack, in the fear that by not doing so you will negatively affect your weight or shape. Obviously there may be times when kitchen scales are essential for baking or cooking, to execute a recipe, and if that's the case give yourself permission to use them for an agreed purpose, and for anything that falls outside of this, remove the battery.

Sunday
Bin the bathroom scales.

This will all feel pretty overwhelming, particularly if these behaviours have been the norm for you for some time. Some of you may be able to bite the bullet and stop using these objects immediately. For others, it may take a little longer and you might find yourself drawn back to using them again. It is important to treat yourself with kindness and not interpret this as another 'failure'. Accept that there are bound to be slip-ups while you unlearn these behaviours. The thoughts and temptations to weigh yourself or to track what you eat may always be there, but it is about getting to a point where you are able to weaken the hold they have over you.

If you find yourself reaching for one of these objects despite the 7-day ditch, stop yourself in your tracks, put the object down and ask yourself:

'Is this object likely to make me feel good about myself?'
'What will this object *actually* tell me?'

Challenge yourself to think about what the object cannot tell you.

'It can't tell me what a good friend I am.'
'It can't tell me how brave I have been supporting my unwell mother.'

It is important to be aware of when your desire to track what you eat, your weight and your body shape becomes a real problem for you. For some patients I see, thoughts about their body can become all-consuming and distressing. They affect their personal, social and working lives. It may take its toll on their mood, and they might even start to experience problems with their physical health as a result. If this is something that rings true for you, it is important to seek support from your family doctor or GP.

Change your outlook

Your beliefs

How we interpret new experiences often stems from deep-rooted beliefs that we hold about ourselves, other people and the world. These may not be immediately obvious to us until a particular situation has brought them to the surface, usually through an emotional response.

Albert Ellis, a psychologist and proponent of the ABC (activating event, belief and consequence) model, challenged the idea that only people or situations (activating events) determine how we feel and act (the consequence) in a given situation.

He proposed a missing link. Rather than an event being directly responsible for how we feel, he suggested that it is our interpretation of a situation, i.e. what we think or **believe**, that ultimately makes us feel and act the way we do.

For instance, if you feel low following an argument with your partner and abruptly end the relationship, rather than directly blaming 'the argument' for how you feel, feeling low may stem from a deep-rooted belief that '*to be in a happy, loving relationship that lasts, you must never argue*'. So when an argument erupts it triggers this irrational belief that might lead you to conclude that the relationship mustn't be a 'happy one', which may see you abruptly end it.

Continuing to hold this irrational belief will undoubtedly continue to affect how you think, feel and act in future relationships. When faced with another activating event (a disagreement or argument – which we all know is part and parcel of even the most loving of relationships), the emotional response of feeling low and the behavioural response of ending the relationship is repeated and strengthened. It may reinforce an idea you hold that you are '*no good at relationships*' or that '*you'll be alone forever*', which can be detrimental to your self-esteem and overall mental wellbeing.

Ellis proposed a form of therapy called rational emotive therapy (RET), which looks to challenge those irrational beliefs and reframe them, or rather look at them differently, and as such develop healthier ways to act.

Meet Megan:

Megan's train is running late. She is on her way to meet her friend for dinner to celebrate her friend getting engaged. She is pacing up and down the platform getting more and more anxious as it becomes increasingly obvious she won't make it on time. She texts her friend apologetically and they come to the conclusion that by the time Megan does make it into town they will have missed the table booking. They take a rain check. Megan feels awful and worries that her friend will not speak to her after all this.

Using the ABC model, I explored Megan's situation with her, the train running late (activating event) that led to her feeling anxious and like an awful friend (consequence). On unpacking this we were able to establish that Megan's emotional response really stemmed from the belief that:

'I can never be late.' 'Being late is disrespectful.'

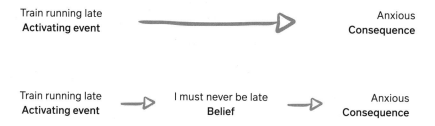

Train running late
Activating event
Anxious
Consequence

Train running late
Activating event
I must never be late
Belief
Anxious
Consequence

Megan was able to think of other situations where she had been late and similarly felt devastated: running late for work when her taxi got held up, or having to help a passer-by in the street and running late for a coffee date as a result.

*We conceded that the problem with these rules or beliefs meant that she held herself to impossibly high standards. By that reckoning, Megan is **never allowed to be late**, even in situations where objectively it is completely out of her control. Because Megan's belief was so fixed, it meant that she could never accept an alternative explanation.*

We agreed that it would be helpful for Megan to express her belief as a preference, an ideal – 'Ideally I would never be late for anything' rather than 'I must never be late' – and to accept that she could not predict that this would always be the case, i.e. that she would never be late.

To help Megan make peace with this and to become more flexible, we reframed how she might alternatively interpret the situation and offered a more rational belief.

While Megan would almost certainly still feel guilty and anxious about being late, we were now able to get her to accept that 'the train being late was not her fault and was out of her control'.

She was able to reframe that her friend was likely to feel 'disappointed' that they wouldn't be celebrating rather than 'annoyed', particularly as it had not been something she had done deliberately.

THE 5 SENSE CHALLENGE:
switching up your
own beliefs

Have you ever thought a person or situation directly affects how you feel? Have you ever considered that it might be your missing link – your interpretation or **belief** about the situation that is at the root of why you feel the way you do?

Next time you find yourself in a situation which feels less than ideal:

1. **ACTIVATING EVENT:** Define what the event is, e.g. train running late.
2. **CONSEQUENCE:** How does it makes you feel? e.g. guilty.
3. **BELIEF:** Consider the missing link. What beliefs have you overridden in this situation that *really* explain why you feel the way you do? e.g. I must never be late.

Notes

....

....

....

....

....

The campsite of beliefs

I developed the 'campsite of beliefs' as a way of thinking about how we might bias the beliefs we hold. Have you ever been convinced something is true and then tried to find other examples of why it must be true in order to prove what you believe?

You might be convinced that your partner is forever dozing off when you talk about work, so you remind them of every occasion they have done so but refuse to recall the countless times when they have been there hanging on your every word.

You might decide to embark on a new diet trend, much to the dismay and concern of your friends around you, who worry that it might cause you more harm than good. To prove your belief that 'this is the right diet for you', you read up all the articles talking about it but only pull out the ones that prove your point, ignoring the others that contradict it, to show them.

Even when there may be evidence or proof that contradicts what you believe, you selectively interpret all the available information in a way that supports your belief. This is what is commonly referred to as confirmation bias.

I know I have been guilty of confirmation bias myself. To convince my husband why I just *have* to buy myself that new handbag, I might pull out every review that says 'This is the bag that every woman needs', and ignore the negative reviews that talk about its cheap material and the problems other buyers have had with it.

What's the problem? By only interpreting and using the information this way, to uphold our own beliefs, we ignore all the objective facts that might be information that is important to us and that may have led to a different outcome.

You may end the relationship on the basis that your partner doesn't listen to you, you might become really unwell as a result of your latest diet fad, and I may buy that handbag only for the strap to snap within the first week.

It is important that next time you find yourself searching for evidence or proof for something you believe, you step back and look at it objectively. Ask yourself whether you are looking at all the information and evidence available to you, or are only sifting out the bits that serve you. Would taking a more balanced view have meant a different outcome? Even if it's not an outcome that you particularly wanted?

Meet Sam:

Sam has a poor track record when it comes to love and holding down a relationship. She finds that she never quite makes it past the first couple of dates before the guys she sees lose interest – at least that is what she assumes happens. She came out of a long-term relationship with her ex-boyfriend Zak a few years ago. Zak was the love of her life. He broke her heart and Sam has struggled to move on since.

On speaking to Sam she came to the conclusion that:

'She was never going to find love' (rule about herself). 'All men were going to cheat on her' (rule about others). 'Love wasn't meant for her' (rule about the world).

This meant that Sam automatically approached each potential suitor defensively. She half-heartedly filled out her online dating profile. She didn't really engage on her dates and refused to let her guard down. When a second date never materialized, rather than consider that it might be down to how she was behaving, she took it as more evidence that 'she was unlovable', that 'all men were going to cheat on her', and that 'love wasn't meant for her'. It became a self-fulfilling prophecy which became stronger and increasingly difficult to shake.

I asked Sam to consider each of her beliefs as tents within a campsite and each peg as evidence for her beliefs that keep the tents secured and fixed to the ground. Her belief (tent) was never able to fly away or be taken down for as long as she continued to find evidence, through unsuccessful date after unsuccessful date (pegs), to keep it in place.

Sam needed to stop finding pegs to secure her beliefs down and to start removing them or placing them elsewhere (in the peg bag), to weaken the hold of the belief (tent) so that she could take the tent down.

In order to do this, she had to accept that she could be wrong. We started to consider why she could be wrong about the fact that she would never be loved. We had a look at the evidence for and against her beliefs.

By getting Sam to consider and accept that she 'didn't really make an active effort on her dates', that 'her boyfriends before her ex didn't cheat', or that she 'was only half-heartedly filling her dating profile', she was able to start loosening the pegs that held down the belief that she was unlovable. As the tent started to take flight, so did Sam's motivation to start helping herself by putting some effort into the dating process. She took the first step by overhauling her dating profile to make sure it captured who she really was.

THE 5 SENSE CHALLENGE:
taking the tent down

Think about your own campsite of beliefs. What beliefs do you hold about different situations? Do you continue to seek out evidence to prove these beliefs right and keep them fixed to the ground? Next time you find yourself thinking negatively, think about the tents and your peg bag. Challenge yourself to think about how you might pull some of those pegs out of the ground and put them back into the bag and weaken the hold that belief (tent) has.

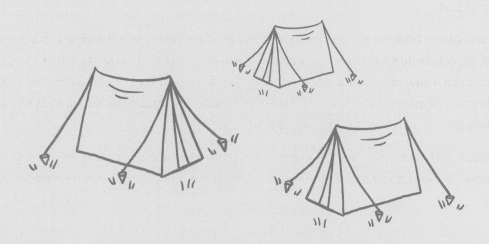

Some of those pegs will be placed firmly into the ground, but by getting used to challenging them, fiddling around and trying to loosen them, you start to weaken the hold they have over you.

Choosing the people you see

The company you keep

The people we surround ourselves with – family, friends and work colleagues – have a huge impact on our mood and mental wellbeing. Social relationships and staying connected have been associated with our ability to regulate and manage stress. If we are feeling stressed, social relationships, particularly those that are able to meet our needs at that time, help us interpret that stress and minimize the impact it has on us. It has also been shown that adults who are more socially connected are healthier and live longer than their more isolated peers. Studies show that if we feel lonely, have fewer social relationships and poor-quality relationships, we are more susceptible to symptoms of depression.

I know when I have woken up in a good mood only to be met with my husband's stonking one, my positivity soon becomes a distant memory. I might try in vain to coax him out of it, to crack a joke only to find that it aggravates him even further. I convince myself that it won't rub off on me, but it is only a matter of time before I get immersed in it myself and subsequently start my day on an equally bad footing.

Similarly, when my daughter bounds into my bedroom excited about an upcoming holiday, her joy can be infectious, and it is impossible to avoid sharing that excitement.

> **If we are feeling stressed, social relationships, particularly those that are able to meet our needs at that time, help us interpret that stress and minimize the impact it has on us.**

For some of us, other people's moods may incite the opposite feeling: when you are feeling low, a close friend's enthusiasm and positivity may in fact accentuate how you are feeling and make you feel worse.

I routinely hear patients offer justifications for the negative people in their life or for the way those around them make them feel. Most of the time they will excuse a partner, friend or family member's behaviour as something they have come to expect from that individual.

'That's just [*insert name*].'

Does doing this (excusing their behaviour) suddenly negate their unacceptable behaviour, regardless of how it makes us feel emotionally?

Ask yourself

Imagine a friend is talking to you about someone in their life who is constantly belittling and criticizing him or her. As an outsider looking on at that situation, what would you say to that friend?

....

....

....

What is it that prevents us from being able to take our own sound advice and avoid similarly getting hurt?

....

....

....

Why are we any less worthy of being treated with respect and dignity?

....

....

....

Often, we can see things with more clarity when a situation is not affecting us directly. We don't have as much to lose and are not as emotionally invested.

THE 5 SENSE CHALLENGE:
the friend litmus test

Think about all the different people you come into contact with each day. This can be anyone from your partner whom you wake up next to, your barista who makes your coffee on a morning or your boss, right through to your friends. Jot each of them down.

You might want to use the log on the next page or fire up the notes section on your phone if you want to be more discreet.

Think about how these people honestly make you *feel*.

Record your wellbeing temperature beside each individual; what colour best reflects your relationship or friendship *overall*, where red is fraught with constant comparisons, catty comments and negativity and blue is positive and infallible.

Use this log as a baseline to come back to when you find yourself in a disagreement with a friend or a work colleague. It can help you to distinguish between '*just a bad day*' and what you have come to expect as *the norm* for that individual.

We are all entitled to our off days; it might be that a friend makes you feel like a red one day but generally the friendship is littered with blues and greens. However, if you find that you are constantly feeling red in a friendship, it is important to evaluate *why* you are holding on to it.

It may sound brutal but it is important to recognize the very real impact that other people can have on your mental wellbeing and to really scrutinize how this relationship *actually* serves you. There is no shame in friendships having an expiry date. We often hold on to friendships for sentimental and nostalgic value and overlook the negative impact they may be having on us.

Person	Role	How did you meet?	How often do you see them?	Overall	🌡️

Meet Charles:

Charles has been friends with Ant for the last 20 years. They met at pre-school and have been firm friends since. They have gone through many firsts together. First fallouts, first parties, first kisses, first girlfriends and first swigs of alcohol. As they got older, Charles couldn't help but feel that Ant had taken a different path to him; after all, they were used to doing things together and agreeing most of the time, so to find themselves at loggerheads constantly was unusual. Charles had a good job, he had just proposed to his long-term girlfriend and was looking forward to buying a house and in time starting a family.

Ant on the other hand was still playing the field, was in a job he hated and still happy come Friday night to spend the weekend boozing. Every week Charles would find himself justifying to Ant why he 'didn't want to go out' and facing the usual onslaught of him 'being a bore' or that he 'had changed'. While Charles initially took it as banter, he became frustrated with the constant need to justify his actions. Ant should just 'get it', right? Over time, he found Ant's approach became more and more aggressive. On several occasions he had turned up post-night-out to Charles's flat, ringing the doorbell during the early hours of the morning and waking up his girlfriend and the neighbours in the process. Charles was struggling to identify the positives in their friendship. He was starting to feel resentment that Ant could not just be happy with what was going on in his life right now.

Charles had tried to confront Ant about his behaviour several times, when he was sober, but Ant refused to hear it and they would end up arguing. In the end, Charles accepted that it was nostalgia that saw him holding on to this friendship – they had been friends for so long, surely that counted for something? But on the other hand, he was no longer getting anything positive from this relationship. Rather than ghost him, Charles was able to explain to Ant how his behaviour was making him feel. It's fair to say Ant didn't take it too well and refused to dial it down or check his behaviour. Charles felt he was left with no choice but to sever all ties. His clarity and Ant's stubbornness in not relenting meant that he no longer had to endure any animosity. While Charles missed the 'old times', he was able to accept that Ant had been in his life for a particular time for a particular reason and that it was normal for certain friendships to run their course. Life without Ant meant that Charles no longer felt on edge every time his phone beeped or rang. He was able to focus on his plans for the future without feeling the need to justify himself or endure a barrage of abuse in the process.

THE 5 SENSE CHALLENGE:
the friendship
spring clean

Imagine opening up your wardrobe; an organized chaos.

There are a handful of trusty items, the **ones you feel comfortable and most yourself in.** These tend to be the ones that make it on to the chair in the corner of your bedroom because you are not quite ready to commit them to a wash – there is one more wear out of them, surely?

Then there are those items pushed to the back of the wardrobe that serve as a reminder of a **different time or a different version** of yourself. The ones you might not fit into or that are outdated, that you hold on to and convince yourself that one day you will get back into them or one day they will come back into fashion.

Finally, there are those items that you pull out **every now and again**, for a particular time or purpose, if you have to go to a stuffy works do for instance, but that make you feel anything but yourself.

Marie Kondo has revolutionized how we look at our wardrobe, forcing us to hold it under a compassionate but critical eye and coining the infamous phrase '*Does this spark joy*?' With this in mind, I want you to throw all your current friendships and relationships on to your hypothetical bed. You are now faced with the challenge of either hanging them back in your hypothetical wardrobe or popping them into a bag beside your door ready to bid farewell. Remember, this is not about culling all friendships and relationships, but about having the confidence to hold them up to scrutiny and to force yourself to evaluate what you are getting from them.

'Spring cleaning' questions:

1. Do I show the best side of myself when I am with this person?
2. Do I find myself having to censor what I say for fear of upsetting this person or them not agreeing with me?
3. If someone I knew was friends with this person, what advice would I give?
4. Do I feel guilt-tripped into spending time with them even when I don't want to?
5. Do I feel emotionally drained after spending time with them?
6. Do they constantly put me down and berate me?
7. Is this person demanding of my time and attention?
8. How do I feel when I get a missed call or text from this friend?
9. Does this friendship feel reciprocal? That is, do we both give 50:50 into it?

It is worth mentioning that across our lifetimes there may be situations that arise, such as a friend going through a break-up, grieving or losing a job, where the ratio may feel more 80:20; similarly there may be times when you experience difficulty and rely more heavily on your friend. This is about stepping back and examining the friendship overall.

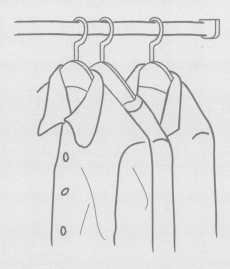

Not quite ready to let it go?

If you want to be able to move forward and resolve the friendship or relationship but this challenge has forced you to acknowledge some difficult truths, then it might be worth having a frank and open conversation with them, particularly if they are a close friend. Jump ahead to Chapter 2, HEAR: 'Just say "no"' and 'Mark of approval' (pages 78 and 86), for some guidance on how to manage a hypercritical friend.

If it's the case that you simply spend too much time with them, you might consider reducing how often you see them and determine if this has any bearing on how you feel and on your wellbeing temperature. While it is unlikely that you will be able to change their particular qualities or personality traits, what you can do is change your own behaviour within that friendship or relationship to ensure you protect your own mental wellbeing.

Chapter 2
HEAR

Hear yourself

Take yourself back to your last high-pressure situation: perhaps a job interview, a driving test or a first date. What was your first thought as you entered that situation? For many, our inner critic makes us think something like: '*You're not going to get the job*' or '*It is going to be a disaster*' or '*They won't fancy you.*' Sound familiar? If so, how did that thought make you feel? Perhaps sick, butterflies in your stomach, a racing heart rate. And how did those feelings make you act? Perhaps you fluffed up on one of the questions, forgot to check your mirrors for that parking manoeuvre or made your excuses and left early. All too often we can find ourselves caught up in the vicious cycle of think, feel, act that leads us to feel overwhelmed. By learning to rationalize and manage our thoughts, we can change how we talk to ourselves, the way we feel and act, and weaken the cycle.

By learning to rationalize and manage our thoughts, we can change how we talk to ourselves, the way we feel and act, and weaken the cycle.

When you think you are 'under threat' (for example, pre-interview nerves) the amygdala (the part of your brain responsible for processing emotions) sends a signal to the hypothalamus (another region of your brain, responsible for communicating with the rest of the body). The hypothalamus communicates with your autonomic nervous system, which is comprised of two parts: your sympathetic nervous system, tasked with initiating your fight-or-flight response, and your parasympathetic nervous system, tasked with calming you down after the threat has been and gone.

Your sympathetic nervous system communicates with your adrenal glands, which triggers the release of adrenaline into your bloodstream. Adrenaline leads to a number of changes within your body which you can feel. It can cause your heart to race faster, which ensures that the blood is getting to where it needs to go – like the muscles in your legs in case you need to make a swift exit. It also makes you breathe faster so you can take as much oxygen on board as possible. Adrenaline also releases blood sugar and fats, further supplying your body with the energy it needs.

If you perceive that you are still under threat – perhaps you step into that interview and your interviewer is scary – the hypothalamus triggers another pathway (the HPA axis) that ultimately leads to the release of cortisol (your stress hormone). This helps to keep you in that constant state of alert. When you feel less threatened, your parasympathetic nervous system is triggered, which supports you in calming down and reduces the stress response.

The way you think about situations, the words you tell yourself, will impact how these systems are triggered and it can *even* affect how you act. That feeling sick ahead of a job interview may have forced you to act less complacent and to put the graft in (fight). Or you might become so overwhelmed with your thoughts and feelings that you avoid putting the work in (flight). Rather than interpreting anxiety ahead of an interview as being a sign that you're not going to get the job, reframe this as excitement at possibly landing your dream job.

Meet Claire:

*Claire is invited on a night out with her friends. Her mind tells her 'I'm not slim enough' **(think)**. She suddenly **feels** anxious; her tummy is tied in knots and she feels a little queasy. Her wellbeing temperature is red. She immediately searches for something to wear **(act)**. Nothing fits. This fuels another cycle of negative thinking, with her mind telling her 'she is fat' and she 'has no self-control' **(think)**. Her tummy ties itself further in knots and her shoulders start to tense **(feel)**.*

Situation: invited on night out with friends

↓

Thought
I'm not slim enough
I'm a bad friend
I have no self-control

Act
Doesn't go on night out
Binge-eats

Mind feels:
Anxious, Guilt

Body feels:
Tense shoulders, Feeling sick

*She decides to do a liquid fast for the next 24 hours in a quest to flatten her tummy **(act)**. Having gone almost 24 hours without food, she starts to feel sick, which worsens those body signals she is already experiencing – stomach in knots and feeling queasy **(feel)**.*

*She decides to avoid going out altogether and sends a text to a friend to apologize **(act)**. Her mind instantly tells her that she is 'a bad friend' and that she 'is worthless' **(think)**. Yet more butterflies in the tummy and feelings of guilt and inadequacy soon follow **(feel)**. She sets up camp in front of the TV and works her way through a pack of biscuits **(act)**. She feels uncomfortable and bloated **(feel)**, which makes her think 'I am fat' or 'I have no self-control' **(think)**.*

Avoiding the night out did little to relieve how Claire was feeling about herself – if anything it fuelled her negative thinking even further. She was left thinking that she had let her friends down, which made her feel even more anxious and guilty, which meant her tummy tied itself in even tighter knots. She subsequently reached for the biscuits as comfort, which made her feel even more guilty and fuelled her thoughts that she had 'no self-control', which meant that she ate even more biscuits and felt even more nauseous. Ultimately Claire found herself caught up in a vicious cycle of thinking, feeling and acting. She felt increasingly overwhelmed and anxious and couldn't see a way out.

I introduced Claire to the concept of mindfulness, to help her take a temporary pause, regroup her thoughts and feel calmer, and to hopefully enable her to act in more positive ways.

The Cambridge Dictionary defines mindfulness as '*the practice of being aware of your body, mind and feelings in the present moment, thought to create a feeling of calm*'. There is a common misconception that mindfulness-based activities are about 'clearing your mind' or ignoring any negative thoughts or feelings, but this is simply not the case. Rather, mindfulness is about accepting these thoughts if they do enter your mind but not dwelling on them, quickly refocusing on the task you are doing rather than allowing yourself to get caught up in that think-feel-act cycle that will just make you feel overwhelmed.

There is some evidence starting to emerge on the beneficial effects mindfulness-based activities and acceptance of present-moment experiences (thoughts, feelings and body sensations) have on our anxiety levels, with some potential promise on its role in treating depression; studies show that patients who learned mindful meditation have demonstrated a better resilience to stressful psychological challenges. Examples of mindfulness-based activities include:

· the body scan: bringing attention to all parts of the body and body sensations in turn
· mindful breathing
· being more aware of daily activities, such as eating without distraction
· gentle exercise, yoga

A simple mindfulness-based technique I routinely recommend to my patients is the 5 sense countdown.

THE 5 SENSE CHALLENGE:
the 5 sense countdown

The 5 sense countdown is about shifting our attention to the present rather than getting caught up in our think-feel-act cycle, which is likely to make us feel more overwhelmed.

Record your wellbeing temperature before starting the exercise.

Find a quiet spot, if you are able to.

Don't worry too much about pushing those negative thoughts away or keeping those uncomfortable feelings at bay. If they enter your mind, acknowledge them, but bring your focus back to the task.

Focus on **5 things that you can SEE** in your immediate environment. Silently take these all in or feel free to say them out loud.

I can see my hair
I can see the birds in the trees
I can see commuters catching a bus
I can see a red car
I can see the thread work in my cardigan

Once you have done this, I want you to focus on the next sense.

4 things that you can HEAR
I can hear the honking of a car horn
I can hear the coughing of a commuter
I can hear the leaves rustling
I can hear someone whistling

3 things that you can SMELL

I can smell the fumes from a nearby exhaust

I can smell the nearby bakery

I can smell the morning mildew

2 things that you can FEEL

I can touch the roughness of my jeans

I can touch my nose

1 thing that you can TASTE

I can taste my mints

Record your wellbeing temperature after the exercise.

Has your temperature come down? Are you feeling less overwhelmed? Do you feel calmer?

This exercise has helped many of my patients take a momentary break from their think-feel-act cycle, reducing feelings of anxiety and helping them think more rationally about how best to act in a given situation.

Faulty thoughts

Faulty thoughts, or 'cognitive distortions' as they are more commonly referred to in the literature, are irrational thinking patterns you might find yourself caught up in that can make you feel negative emotions and act in less than desirable ways.

We can all experience these irrational thoughts in varying degrees and it can affect some of us more negatively than others. It is helpful to be aware of the most common types of 'faulty thought', as learning to spot them can help you stop the thought in its tracks, challenge it and mitigate how it might then make you feel or go on to act. We will take a look at how you might challenge or reframe these thoughts a little later.

Types of faulty thoughts

Fortune-telling

'I will not learn everything in time.'

'I'm going to be rubbish at it anyway.'

Have you ever told yourself that you can't do something before you have even given it a go? Do you predict how it will turn out and get so bogged down with what you think might happen that you are not able to enjoy the process of getting there? This is fortune-telling – where you jump to (negative) conclusions about how a situation might pan out.

Next time you catch yourself fortune-telling, think about what evidence you have that whatever you think will happen is going to. Often the only evidence you have is your inner critic or those faulty thoughts.

Remind yourself that this is a faulty thought, that you can't possibly know what will happen in the future, and that getting lost in the 'what might happen' means that you're not able to enjoy the present-moment experience.

Over-generalizing

'I failed that one time therefore I will always fail.'

'My niece cried when I held her, therefore all babies will cry when I hold them.'

Have you ever had one bad experience and have now become convinced that this will always happen? You are more cautious about entering similar situations, possibly even avoidant, for the fear of a similar negative experience playing out?

Next time you catch yourself over-generalizing, remind yourself that just because something has happened once, it doesn't mean it will always happen.

Remind yourself that this is a faulty thought and that getting lost in the 'it will happen again' will get in the way of you being able to enjoy future experiences. Reflect on the 'bad' experience and, rather than assume it will happen again, think about what measures you can put in place to prepare yourself for the next time. Do you need to do more prep work? Do you need to read up on the umpteen reasons why a baby might cry?

Mind-reading

'Everyone is thinking that I can't do this.'

'They didn't ring me back, they must be ignoring me.'

Have you ever been convinced that you know what people are thinking of you even before they have opened their mouth to speak? You assume they think a certain way about you, often negatively, so you change the way you think, feel and act in response. You might talk yourself out of doing something or struggle to give something 100% because of what you believe they think of you. You jump to a (negative) conclusion.

Next time you find yourself mind-reading, tell yourself that you can't possibly know what everyone thinks of you. Remind yourself that this is a faulty thought and that your perception of what this person might not even think of you is getting in the way of you being able to experience something potentially quite positive. Rationally tell yourself that 'they haven't actually told me that I am [insert chosen adjective]' and move on.

Personalization

'They never seem to be in when I pop round, it must be me.'

Have you ever claimed responsibility when something doesn't go to plan or doesn't quite pan out the way you expected, when there may be a number of reasons to explain it? Do you automatically assume that it has something to do with you or with something you have done?

Next time you find yourself personalizing, remind yourself that this is a faulty thought. Tell yourself that you can't be held responsible for the outcome of certain events or for how people respond. Think about how the burden of continuing to think you are responsible for something when you are not will impact on future situations. It might mean that you avoid certain situations because you believe you cause or bring on an undesired outcome.

Filtering

'Despite passing the exam, I can't help but think about the answers I didn't get right.'

Have you ever been in a situation where you lose sight of the positives and just focus on the negatives? It can be something that you dwell on repeatedly; you punish yourself and you struggle to enjoy any form of success because you are always blindsided by the things that you didn't get right or achieve.

Next time you find yourself filtering, remind yourself that this is a faulty thought. Ask yourself whether you are looking at the whole picture or whether you have just focused in on one detail that happens to be negative. Are you then basing how you feel about that one experience on that one detail? What are the positives that you can see? Make sure that you are giving those equal attention. Challenge yourself to jot down the negatives and the positives.

Catastrophizing

'My partner has broken up with me, I will be single for ever.'

'I've just cut my finger on a sheet of paper, it will bleed for ever.'

Have you ever exaggerated an already negative situation by fearing the absolute worst will happen and blowing it way out of proportion? You experience something negative but build it up in your mind to being something far bigger than it should be.

Next time you find yourself catastrophizing, remind yourself that this is a faulty thought. Be compassionate and acknowledge the experience as being an unpleasant one – 'it's not nice that my boyfriend has broken up with me', 'it's not ideal getting a paper cut' – but accept that these unpleasant things are a part of life. What you do have control over is how much you blow it out of proportion and make it more unpleasant than it needs to be. If you do find yourself catastrophizing, consider what you may actually be worried about: 'My ex has made me feel really unlovable', 'I'm worried that I've cut myself quite deeply.'

Ask yourself how likely the worst possible outcome is to happen. Challenge yourself to think: What if it did happen? How could you cope? Who or what could you draw upon to help support you?

Labelling

'Putting together this flatpack is no good, I'm no good.'

'I've failed that exam, I'm a failure.'

'They can't even listen to one simple instruction, they are useless.'

Have you ever completed a task or found yourself in a situation that might be difficult, and you assume and conclude very quickly that it must be something to do with you and go on to give yourself a disparaging label? How about when someone does something you don't approve of, do you label them rather than view their behaviour as being less than desirable? By labelling yourself rather than seeing the flatpack instructions as no good or accepting that the exam was difficult, you run the risk of damaging your self-esteem. Similarly by labelling someone as useless, you do little to instil confidence in them and their abilities.

Next time you find yourself on the brink of labelling yourself or someone else, ask yourself: what behaviour am I really labelling here? Be compassionate to yourself or them and provide an alternative, more reflective explanation.

'I am not useless. Those flatpack instructions are difficult to make sense of so it is unsurprising that I have found it difficult to put together.'

'Yes, I've failed that exam but the exam was really difficult, which meant that my answers weren't as strong.'

'They haven't listened to what I am saying, maybe I need to be clearer in communicating what I want.'

Black-and-white (or all-or-nothing) thinking
'I need to be the perfect mum. I need to know everything or I needn't bother at all.'

'I either eat healthily or I binge-eat junk.'

Have you ever been black-and-white in the way you have looked at things – there is no grey area, no middle ground? Either you are this or you are that? Either you do something or you don't bother doing it at all? If someone lets you down once, they will do it again. People, places or objects are either good or bad, right or wrong. You perceive others or situations as polarized. Looking at things as black-and-white as this, or being all-or-nothing with your thinking, might mean that you stop opening yourself up to new experiences and potentially stifle any self-growth. You have already decided how something will be or how a situation might pan out, so you write it off.

Next time you find yourself looking at situations as black or white, ask yourself whether you are missing any of the grey areas. Be compassionate with yourself. If you are telling yourself you need to know everything (that there is to being a mum) or you 'may as well not bother', reframe this by telling yourself that you can't possibly know everything there is to know and that there will be times you will make a mistake and that is OK.

The 'shoulds' and the 'if onlys'

'I should have done x and maybe I would have got the job.'

'I should have called her back, if I had then maybe we would still be friends.'

Have you ever held yourself ransom to something you think you should have done? When something happens you tell yourself that if only you had done things differently – the 'I should have' – then maybe the outcome would have been different, more desirable. By ruminating over the 'shoulds' or 'if onlys' you become embroiled in a cycle of anger, self-loathing or feeling guilty for getting yourself into the situation you are now in. And the result? It doesn't achieve anything.

Next time you find yourself reflecting on the 'shoulds' or 'if onlys', stop the thought in its tracks. Remind yourself that this is a faulty thought. You can't possibly know whether that hypothetical scenario you play out in your mind will come to fruition in the way you imagine, and by convincing yourself it will do, you just torture yourself in the process. Accept that this is the outcome, however uncomfortable it might feel, and work towards thinking about how you can move forward – what can you proactively do differently next time to avoid the undesired outcome from happening again?

Minimizing

'It was nothing.'

'It's nothing to be proud of – the questions I got right were simple enough.'

Have you ever downplayed your achievements? Can you never truly enjoy your successes because you minimize them? Often we see minimization coexist with magnification; you magnify and hone in on the negatives of a situation, discounting or minimizing any positives that may have come from it.

Next time you find yourself downplaying an achievement, stop your thought in its tracks. Remind yourself that this is a faulty thought. Ask yourself whether you are giving more importance to the negative. Challenge yourself to write down the positives from a situation and, crucially, allow yourself to celebrate them or be self-congratulatory.

'They're right, I did a good job there.'

'Yes, I may have got some things wrong, but look at all the things I have got right.'

By celebrating these successes, you bolster your self-confidence and self-esteem and motivate yourself to keep doing what you are doing.

Emotional reasoning

'I feel fat, therefore I must be fat.'

'I feel stupid, therefore I am stupid.'

Have you ever experienced an emotion and then gone on to embody it, so that it becomes your identity? You feel it, therefore you are it. You feel it, therefore it must be true. This can go on to impact how you think, feel and act based on something for which you had very little evidence to begin with. You might cover up, turn down social invites because you feel and believe yourself to be fat. You might not pipe up during a dinner party debate because you feel and believe you are stupid.

Next time you find yourself drawing a conclusion based on how you feel, remind yourself that this is a faulty thought. Be compassionate and tell yourself that 'just because you feel a certain way doesn't mean that it is true or that it defines you'. Feeling is not fact.

Ask yourself

To help you challenge your faulty thoughts, use this reframe tool.

Tick the *faulty thought* that you think you are experiencing:

I am fortune-telling ☐   I am labelling ☐

I am over-generalizing ☐   I am black-and-white (all-or-nothing)

I am mind-reading ☐   thinking ☐

I am personalizing ☐   I am using 'shoulds' and 'if onlys' ☐

I am jumping to conclusions ☐   I am minimizing ☐

I am filtering ☐   I am emotionally reasoning ☐

I am catastrophizing ☐

What evidence do you have that this thought is right?

....

....

....

What evidence is there that you may be wrong?

....

....

....

Are you basing this thought on your opinion or is this based on something you know to be true?

....

....

....

What is continuing to think this way likely to do?

....

....

....

What would you tell a friend who shared these thoughts with you?

....

....

....

Is there another way of reframing this thought?

....

....

....

What has reframing this thought allowed you to do differently?

....

....

....

Just say 'no'

Ever talked yourself out of a workout because you weren't feeling up to it? What about taking sick leave when you were bedridden with the flu? There are certain situations where you feel more comfortable just saying 'no', but other times when you ignore signs of burnout and soldier on regardless. Feeling stressed and overwhelmed at home or the workplace and being busy have become badges of honour. But at what cost? Is being busy but running yourself ragged in the process *really* worth it?

If you are someone who fears saying 'no', why is this? I know personally, when I say 'no', I conjure up this idea that '*I am not being helpful*', '*I'm being selfish*', or '*I don't care*'.

Saying 'yes', for many of us, is far less complicated, even if at times this comes at the expense of our own preferences or wellbeing.

'Yes, I will come on that night out' – even if it means sacrificing the only evening I have had to myself in months.

'Yes, I will run that project' – even though I am still working on the other one that you gave me less than 24 hours ago.

'Yes, I will go on that date with you' – because I don't want to be mean.

Saying 'yes' means acceptance from others; it means not letting anyone down. However, saying 'yes' when you really mean 'no' can breed resentment, lead you to feel overwhelmed and negatively impact your mental wellbeing. This is by no means an open invitation to go round saying 'no' to every opportunity or request that comes your way. Rather, this is about valuing yourself, your time and your wellbeing *more*; at the very least to say '*I'll think about it*'.

Ask yourself

Imagine you are preparing for an upcoming holiday. You have decided the destination. You've got the dates booked. Travel and accommodation are sorted. You know exactly how long you are going for and who you are going with. You have chosen this destination for a particular reason (weather, activities, culture, food), and the perks that come with the package you have booked. Imagine you turn up at the airport. Your flight is ready to board, so you head towards the departure gate. Someone stops you and says:

'You have to go here [insert alternative destination] instead.'

What do you say?

....

....

....

....

Imagine an alternative scenario. You and your partner decide to be a little more spontaneous. You pack a weekend bag and meet at the airport. You're not quite sure where you want to go but hope that you will be inspired when you look at the departures board. That same person approaches you and says:

'You have to go here [insert destination].'

What would you say now?

....

....

....

....

I imagine your answers might well be different for each of the scenarios, but why is this?

In the first scenario, you are clear on your goal – '*I want to go to [insert chosen holiday destination]*.' You have prepared yourself mentally – '*I can't wait until I am on that beach or on those slopes*' – and prepared practically, packing swimwear or ski wear depending. You know that you have booked a specific flight and accommodation the other side and *that* flight is the one you need to get on to enjoy said holiday. Because you are clear on your goals, have made steps to prepare and know your final destination, saying 'no' feels easier, there is no hesitation.

However, in the second scenario, you had none of the certainty of the above, you knew you wanted to go away, you weren't sure where you wanted to go, or why, so you were easily swayed into saying 'yes', even if you felt more than a little apprehensive about it.

While there may be an initial excitement in saying 'yes', the other side could mean a different story – the break could end up being far from relaxing, the accommodation a dive, and you may not have packed the right attire. All of which can see you resenting the person who got you to say 'yes'.

This exercise demonstrates how important it is to be clear in your own mind about what you want to get out of your life and from your friendships and relationships, so that when these get called into question, or another experience or opportunity presents itself, you can really think about whether this serves what is important to you and, if it doesn't, be assertive and confident in being able to communicate that.

'*No, I won't go on that flight because I am looking forward to my break here and getting some sun.*'

Determining what's important and knowing when to say 'no'

Breeding resentment

Ever feel that you are forced into a situation where you feel you have no choice but to say 'yes'? You can end up resenting the person who has asked you to carry out the said task, whether it is to join them on that night out (when all you wanted was an early night) or to help them with their workload before even being able to tackle your own.

It is important to remember that when someone asks whether you can do something, they are effectively giving you a choice. '*Can you do* x or y' is completely different from '*Do* x and y.'

Meet Dave:

Dave works for an events company. It is their busiest time of year, the festive period. He is working every hour God sends at the moment. He accepts that this is the nature of his job, which makes him even more precious about his downtime, of which he has very little at the moment.

One of Dave's rare days off rolls around and his friend wastes no opportunity in asking Dave whether he wants to come out with all the other lads for a 'night out, just like old times'. Dave can't think of anything worse. 'Please, when was the last time we were all out together?', 'You have to come,' his friend pleads. Dave feels put on the spot. He has his internal 'no' in a spin. Dave feels he would be 'letting his friend down' and that he 'would be a bad sport' if he didn't go.

We reflected on what was important to Dave personally, socially and from a working perspective: Right now? Next week? Next year?

Dave's importance list:

Personal goals
At the moment: *being happy, being able to do things that make me happy, such as lounging on the sofa watching Netflix, exercising.*
Next week: *meeting a partner, being able to learn to dance.*
Next year: *getting married, being a dad, being able to go part-time.*

Social goals
At the moment*: honesty, openness, trust within current friendships, avoiding heavy nights out.*
Next week*: being able to go out with friends once work lets up.*
Next year*: organizing a friend's stag.*

Working goals
At the moment*: getting through the festive period.*
Next week*: getting the diary in check for the next calendar year.*
Next year*: would like to get promoted.*

*At the moment, Dave's main focus is getting through the festive period and ensuring he nails the events they have coming up **(working; at the moment)**.*

*He also recognizes that his downtime is just as important; an opportunity to just unwind in front of the TV or thrash it out at the gym **(personally; at the moment)**.*

*Socially it is important for him to be surrounded by friends that he can trust and be open with **(socially; at the moment)**.*

*Going out didn't serve Dave or his goals **right now**. Valuing honesty and openness within his friendships meant that he could share just how stressed he was feeling and that a night out was the last thing on his mind. Because Dave had such clear goals (the things that were important for him to achieve) in all aspects of his life, he felt confident and more empowered to say 'no' and let go of the guilt that he would otherwise be consumed by.*

THE 5 SENSE CHALLENGE:
the importance list

In your personal, social and working life, what is important to you, at the moment, next week and next year?

Often we say 'yes' to things because we are not sure of our own journey, so it feels easier to jump on the next outbound flight and hope that it takes us somewhere half decent.

By being certain of what is important to you, you can make sure everything you agree to is taking you in a direction that brings you closer to that.

Ask yourself, does what *x* is asking me to do bring me closer to what is important on my list? If the answer is 'no', then think carefully about the reasons why you feel compelled to say 'yes', and have the confidence at the very least to say '*I'll think about it*'.

Personal goals	Social goals	Working goals
At the moment:	At the moment:	At the moment:
....	....	....
....	....	....
Next week:	Next week:	Next week:
....	....	....
....	....	....
Next year:	Next year:	Next year:
....	....	....
....	....	....

It is important to be mindful that there may be times when we are asked to do something that we would rather say 'no' to, like turning up to work or chairing that meeting, but we know that it will serve us in the long run or enable us to meet those distant goals.

THE 5 SENSE CHALLENGE:
saying 'no' checklist

Next time you are on the receiving end of a request, run through the following questions.

Is this something that is on my **importance list**? Yes/No

Do I **want** to do this? Yes/No

Do I have **time** to do this? Yes/No

If the answer to all of the above questions is 'no', then be bold and **politely decline**.

Avoid overcomplicated explanations and grovelling apologies that will likely just compound any guilt you might feel for 'letting anyone down'.

Be honest. If you have other commitments, let them know that what they are asking of you is likely to clash with those.

To **avoid repeated requests**, let that person know that if your circumstances change and you are able to take on what they ask of you, then you will get in touch with them. This nips in the bud any chance of them coming back to you with the same request.

Mark of approval

Have you ever been guilty of seeking other people's approval to validate something that you have done? Whether it is seeking approval from family and friends, or vying for acceptance at work? It is always nice to hear that you're doing a good job and that what you have to offer is valuable, but at what cost?

By placing others' opinions above our own, what we are saying is, '*I need you to tell me what I am doing is good enough or worthwhile*', which can be damaging to our self-esteem. Suddenly we become dependent on what *other people* say to feel good.

Regaining control

Rather than putting it on to others to decide how you feel in any given moment or over a prolonged period of time, you need to reclaim that control. By being able to cultivate your own self-assurance, you place less value on gaining other people's approval and on how that approval affects you. If someone does turn around and disagree with you, you observe the difference in opinion but it doesn't completely floor you in the way that it would otherwise have done.

Quicksand – self-esteem and the foundations we lay

Bring your attention to the picture below: on the left is a picture of a house on a bed of quicksand. The house depicts your self-esteem and the sand reflects the often changing landscape of other people's approval. Your house (self-esteem) tries to lay down some solid foundations but because of the unpredictability and uncertainty of the land below, it struggles to do so. Your self-esteem is vulnerable and could come crashing down at any moment.

Self-esteem   Self-esteem

   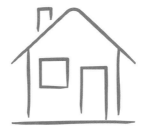

Needing other   Not needing
people's approval   approval

On the right-hand side is another house, this time with solid foundations. This represents what happens when you have a clear understanding of self, your needs and your abilities. You rely less on needing to seek approval from other people. Because of this, your foundation is solid and your self-esteem less fragile.

There could be a number of reasons why someone does not like what you are doing. If what you are doing does not cause you or anyone else any direct harm, then what's the problem? More often than not, disapproval can tell you more about the other person than it does about you. We all have different early life experiences that shape how we approach future ones.

We all have different values, things that are important to us. You might decide that you don't like certain names because they remind you of an ex. You may disapprove of your partner's drinking because you have a family member in the grips of alcoholism. In the example on the following page, Kate might not like Jenna dressing alternatively because it draws attention to them both when they are out together and she struggles with her own body image.

Anything you do has the potential to be met with disapproval from others. You can't control every possible response that may come your way over something you choose or don't choose to do. When we seek external validation, our decision to celebrate becomes dependent on someone else's measure of success, rather than our own.

Meet Jenna:

Jenna has been with her girlfriend for a couple of years. They are pretty happy but Jenna describes always feeling like she is walking on eggshells where Kate is concerned. Kate joked about the fact that Jenna had 'no dress sense' when they first met and it has remained a favourite dinner party story even a couple of years down the line. While Jenna initially found it funny, she is starting to struggle with being the butt of everyone's jokes.

Jenna's dress sense has always been what you would call 'alternative'. She used to enjoy dressing up and used to feel confident in whatever she managed to throw together. There was only so much Jenna could put up with in terms of the eye rolls or the 'You're not wearing that again' or the vigorous head shakes from Kate whenever she presented herself ahead of a day out. As Jenna has started to dress a bit more conservatively, Kate seems more approving of her choices. Despite this, Jenna has never felt more lost and under-confident. She has no idea of who she is any more. The joy she once felt from getting herself dressed up is replaced with a 'nervous anticipation' of whether 'Kate will approve'. When she does approve, Jenna feels temporarily lifted, but when she doesn't it knocks her for six; she feels her self-esteem ebbing away.

Jenna epitomizes this idea of needing the approval and acceptance of others to feel worthy. While it gave Jenna a temporary lift to know that Kate liked what she was wearing, it came at the expense of her ability to express her identity. By Jenna grounding her self-esteem on Kate's approval, it meant that she never knew quite how she should be feeling about herself and what she was capable of. If Kate told her that she looked good, she must look good. If Kate told her she didn't, then she didn't.

Working with Jenna, we established that she had always had a good sense of who she was, what she liked and a confidence to express herself before she met Kate and started their relationship. She would have rated her wellbeing temperature at a respectable green or yellow. Meeting Kate, she knew how opinionated she could get over something as trivial (to Jenna at least) as what she was wearing. The fear of judgement made her feel uncomfortable. She was desperate for Kate to be proud standing by her, so she started to change what she was wearing. She found that when Kate didn't approve of her outfit, her wellbeing temperature pushed up to an orange/red, but when Kate did like what she was wearing, this went down to a green or even blue. The resentment she built towards Kate over time meant that her wellbeing temperature was at an all-time high. She became overwhelmed whenever she went shopping (something she used to enjoy) at the prospect of second-guessing every outfit purchase . . . 'Would Kate like it?'

THE 5 SENSE CHALLENGE:
the approval game

Next time you find yourself seeking approval from someone or second-guessing whether you should or shouldn't do something for fear of how they might react, use the approval log below to jot down your thoughts.

The need for approval may be triggered by anything – nothing is too trivial, whether it is debating if a partner will or won't like a new outfit choice, or deciding whether you're cut out to go for that promotion at work.

Decision that needs to be made; what would I like to do	Need approval because	Need approval from	If I don't get approval	If I get approval	In the long term makes me feel
Meeting a partner's family for the first time. Putting on an outfit and asking my partner what they think.	Need help deciding whether it is the right outfit to wear.	My partner and ultimately my partner's family.	Then I will feel less confident. If my partner doesn't like it, then neither will my partner's family and maybe they won't like me.	I will feel temporarily happy. If my partner likes it then surely my partner's family will too.	Resentful. Why can't they just like whatever I put on?

First and foremost, decide what you want to do. Sounds like a bit of an alien concept, doesn't it?

....

....

....

Think about why you need to seek approval and from who?

....

....

....

What happens if you don't get their approval? And, if you do?

....

....

....

In the long term, how does continuing to need their approval make you feel?

....

....

....

THE 5 SENSE CHALLENGE:
taking back control

Think about what activities you do on a weekly basis and list these below the relevant subsection: personal, social or work.

Record your wellbeing temperature for each activity. With a critical eye, determine whether this is something you do for *yourself* or for *someone else*.

Personal: include things like self-care, grooming, foods you eat, how regularly you exercise, what time you go to bed, interests and hobbies.

*For me/for someone else . . .
*For me/for someone else . . .
*For me/for someone else . . .

Social: include the people you hang out with, relationships, places you go to eat/drink.

*For me/for someone else . . .
*For me/for someone else . . .
*For me/for someone else . . .

Work: the job you are in, working overtime, promotion, taking on another task.

*For me/for someone else . . .
*For me/for someone else . . .
*For me/for someone else . . .

For the activities that routinely see you in the red, determine whether these align with your importance list.

*delete as appropriate

You might not like the fact that you have to work overtime (next week) but you know it has to be done to make sure you save enough money so you can afford to pay off your wedding and honeymoon (next year).

If the RED activities do not serve you, consider whether these need to be done at all. What purpose do they serve, other than as a vehicle to gain someone else's approval?

Start to phase them out. If there are several types of red activity, you may choose to start phasing out one type of red activity at a time. If it is something that you do every day, you may start by dropping how often you do it rather than going cold turkey. You might drop it down to 6 times a week, then 5, and so forth. This may feel overwhelming to begin with, particularly if it is something you have done to keep someone else happy. But over time this might start to feel rather liberating, as your wellbeing temperature in the day cools and you have fewer activities to contend with.

Start to hear compliments

When your boss says you've done a good job, do you find that you struggle to accept the praise? Or do you get bashful when someone comments on your new top? Naturally the self-deprecating comments may follow:

'It was nothing, just doing my job.' 'Thanks, I got it in the sale.' 'This old thing?'

There is some discomfort in being seen to be taking praise: *'Will they think I am arrogant if I agree that my top looks nice?'* or *'Will my boss worry I will become complacent if I accept this as a job well done?'*

How can we impart equal attention to any positive praise that comes our way and start accepting it unapologetically?

Meet Gemma:

Gemma is a personal trainer. She lives and breathes Lycra. Moving from client to client, and with meetings and catch-ups in between, there seems little point in bringing along a separate outfit to get changed into, just for her journey home. Gemma isn't used to people complimenting her outfit; after all, it's practical and essentially her uniform. Come the weekend, once her morning workout is done and dusted, she loves nothing more than giving the other side of her wardrobe a workout and experimenting with makeup. Gemma is still conscious that for a lot of people Lycra is her identity, so being seen out of it is like spotting a schoolteacher out in their 'normal clothes' – it's a bit of an alien concept.

Gemma is off to a baby shower this afternoon, along with some of her friends. She pops on a floral tea dress, a leather jacket and some biker boots.

'You look amazing, Gem,' shrieks one of her friends as she turns up to the venue.

'I had a lie-in so had next to no time to get ready – I look a state', she replies, laughing off the compliment.

'Love the dress,' another friend pipes up.

'What, this thing, I got it in the sale last week during my lunch break. I'm still not sure about it if I'm honest, but it will do.'

Gemma pulls down at the hem of her dress awkwardly and she follows her friends over to the table where their expecting friend is sitting.

She told me that she finds taking compliments like these difficult. Her worry was that people would think she was too muscular to be in a dress. We spoke about the manner in which Gemma responded to her friends' compliments. We conceded that *her excusing her appearance as having 'just-got-out-of-bed' and as 'only having got the dress in the sale' meant that she 'got in there first', before the anticipated cutting remarks about her appearance, even though Gemma had not a shred of evidence that this would be the case. Remember the 'mind-reading' from page 70.*

We spoke about the compliments that Gemma received – the 'you look amazing' and 'great dress'. She felt they were just saying that to be nice and they didn't mean it.

We reflected on whether Gemma's low self-esteem meant that she was unable to hear or accept the praise that came her way and, even more crucially, believe it.

'If I don't think I look good, I just don't believe that anybody else would think I do' – classic black-and-white thinking (see page 73).

Gemma's self-deprecation meant that she never truly felt able to celebrate her individual success and reflected how little she felt about herself. She agreed that she would be more likely to readily accept failure or criticism than she would a compliment. We reflected on how that might feel over time, to continue to internalize the negatives and push away the positives that came her way. While she could be forgiven for being humble, ultimately she was telling herself that she 'is not worthy of this praise'. Repeating this message to herself over time reinforces it and may see her believe it.

Ever thought about how rejecting a compliment from the 'complimenter' might make them feel? For instance, if a partner's attempts to tell you what a wonderful person you are are consistently met with a 'You don't mean that' or 'You're only saying that to be nice', they may be rendered powerless to say anything.

This might mean they feel less confident in giving praise and compliments because doing so can be an exhausting and awkward process of resistance by you and reassurance by them. The lack of praise that follows thereafter might unintentionally compound your low self-esteem: 'They have stopped telling me I am great, therefore I mustn't be.'

Ask yourself

Think about the last time that someone paid you a compliment or showered you with praise. How did you respond?

....

....

....

....

How did hearing the compliment make you feel? *Record your wellbeing temperature.*

....

....

....

....

Do you respond differently depending on who the 'praiser' is? Or is your response the same regardless?

....

....

....

....

Are you someone who is more likely to take on board the negatives that are said about you or your achievements than the positives?

....

....

....

....

If you are someone who finds praise difficult, what is your fear in accepting praise or a compliment?

....

....

....

....

THE 5 SENSE CHALLENGE:
celebrating small wins

If you are someone who struggles with praise, in order to be able to genuinely accept compliments from others, you need to fundamentally believe you are worthy of praise. For a lot of us, being self-critical comes more naturally than the skill of being celebratory of our achievements. I advocate the practice of celebrating small wins daily as part of the antidote to this.

Being able to acknowledge when you have done a good job can not only help improve your confidence but is also a great motivational tool to help spur you on to continue to meet your personal and professional goals, whatever they may be.

Set aside 5–10 minutes each day to celebrate your small wins from the day. This might feel a little overwhelming to begin with, but will become easier with practice. You might like to use this framework:

I am proud of myself for . . .
I was able to achieve . . .
I helped someone . . .

Ensure that you set a reminder on your phone or your calendar; commit to it as you would any other appointment or meeting.

Understanding your response to praise

For each compliment you receive in a given day, tally your response to it under one of the sub-categories below.

Reaction:	Ignore/ change the subject	Laugh it off	'Thanks'	Compliment back	Change the subject	Reject/ downplay yourself

Next, tally your *reason* for responding in the way that you did. What did you fear from accepting the praise?

Why do you fear praise?

Fear:	Being arrogant	Becoming complacent	It's not true – they're just being nice	They are just after something	They want me to compliment them back

THE 5 SENSE CHALLENGE:
the compliment stepladder

If you struggle with receiving compliments, the compliment stepladder will gradually expose you to this fear and work towards feeling more comfortable in accepting them.

Repeat each step until your wellbeing temperature is either blue or green before moving on to the next.

If you remain in that situation (or step) long enough, your anxiety levels will start to reduce. This is explained psychologically by the habituation theory, where continuing to be exposed to a fearful stimulus will naturally reduce the fear response. There is some thinking that being repeatedly faced with a stimulus changes its impact on us; the more familiar we become with it, the less of a threat we see it as.

To give yourself the best chance of achieving success at each step, make sure you stay in each situation long enough to notice a reduction in your anxiety.

Practise, practise, practise. The more you repeat each step, the quicker you will habituate to it.

Resist the urge to jump steps. For instance, if you are still scoring reds and oranges with step 1, don't jump ahead to step 2 where you are forced to verbally acknowledge a compliment. By doing this you may set yourself up to fail, because you may become so overwhelmed with anxiety that you struggle to get back on the ladder. By avoiding the feared situation, you ultimately heighten and reinforce your anxiety.

Step 1: Resist the urge to ignore the compliment or change the topic of conversation. Smile or nod to acknowledge that you have heard the compliment.

Step 2: Say something back to show you have heard the compliment, even a simple 'thanks'.

Step 3: Share with that person how receiving the compliment has made you feel. 'Thanks, I'm glad you enjoyed it' or 'Thanks, you've made my day'.

Step 4: Give a compliment back. 'Thanks, I worked really hard on that. Your input really helped.'

Each week, reflect on where you are on the compliment stepladder. As you start to move up the ladder, think about how learning to accept compliments has made you think, feel and act. I bet within a few weeks you'll feel more confident, stand a little taller and even find that you pay yourself a compliment from time to time.

Ensure that you set a reminder on your phone or your calendar; commit to it as you would any other appointment or meeting.

Meet Edie:

Edie works at a national newspaper as a features writer. She has been in the job for the last 5 years and is desperate to make senior editor. She loves her job but always dreads submitting her article for review, in anticipation of the sea of red pen.

'I like the direction of this piece but I am worried you're not sharing enough of this person's journey', remarks one.

'Great start, but can you clarify what is the subject's view of what you have written here?' reads another.

Edie feels defeated. Overlooks the positive 'great start' and hones in on the criticism that follows (filtering, page 71). Edie doesn't deal with criticism well. She has read her piece. Her partner (who doesn't work in press) gave her a thumbs-up, as did a handful of her friends pre-submission, so she can't understand her boss's problem.

Concluding that this is more her boss's issue rather than anything to do with her piece, she resubmits it back immediately without so much as making a correction.

'Have you responded to my previous notes?' her boss pings back.

I got Edie to think about what her boss was really trying to communicate to her.

'She thinks I am not good enough.' 'She thinks I am ridiculous.' 'She thinks I don't know how to write', she answered defensively.

I challenged Edie to think about how true her thoughts were. Edie conceded that because her articles were always 'red-penned', this was proof if ever she needed it that her boss thought she was useless.

I asked Edie how she felt when she re-sent the unchanged article back to her boss. She remarked that she was fuming, and rated her wellbeing temperature as a red.

I challenged Edie to think about **why** her boss might be 'criticizing' her work. After a bit of time she offered . . .

'Because she wants to sell papers.' 'Because she wants a good story.' 'To maintain the reputation of the paper.'

I asked Edie why writing this article and 'getting it right' might be important to her.

'Because I want to write a good story.' 'Because I want to be a reputable journalist.'

And . . . 'I want to earn my stripes to become a senior editor one day', she added.

We reflected that fundamentally, Edie's and her features director's goals were the same.

By acknowledging this, Edie was able to see the criticism as leading towards her intended goals.

Taking criticism on the chin

Response to criticism

If you are someone who struggles with negative feedback or criticism, you might find yourself responding in a number of different ways:

- You may be upset by what someone has said to you.
- You may believe the criticism as 'truth'.
- You may get angry.
- You may get defensive and shut yourself off.

Making sense of criticism

While it wasn't nice for Edie to hear that her boss wasn't 100% happy with her piece, she could see (once she had calmed down!) that the initial criticism offered of *needing to share more of the person's journey'* was reasonable and gave her something to work with (helpful).

However, if after resubmitting her piece unedited, Edie's boss pinged back *'You're ridiculous'* or *'You never respond to my suggestions'*, *this* feedback is less helpful. In this situation, her boss's criticism labels Edie as the problem rather than her actions (ridiculous for not submitting). It also overgeneralizes that Edie always ignores suggestions when this might not be the case.

Ask yourself

How do you respond when you are faced with criticism?

....

....

Next time you find yourself on the receiving end of criticism, ask yourself:
Who is criticizing you? Is it a friend, family member, colleague or a troll online?

....

....

Step back objectively and consider why this person might be criticizing you.

....

....

Think about whether you have a shared goal.

....

....

Has the 'criticizer' shared constructive ideas on what you can change?

....

....

Has the 'criticizer' labelled you rather than your actions?

....

....

What do you think they are actually trying to communicate?

....

....

How do you feel about the criticism? *Record your wellbeing temperature.*

....

....

Crucially, how do you then go on to act?

....

....

Dealing with criticism

If you've determined that the criticism was not 'constructive criticism' and was simply offensive, disregard it. Tell yourself that there was no purpose to this criticism other than to hurt you. The criticizer has not offered you the opportunity to grow or develop from what they have said. In these situations, someone else's criticism may have very little to do with you and a lot to do with them. Ever had a bad day and taken it out on your nearest and dearest or a colleague in the shared office? It might be that someone's bad day, their receipt of bad news or their own insecurities, coupled with your proximity to them, made you a convenient scapegoat. While not entirely fair, it enables you to consider an alternative argument to criticism or trolling that seems unjust, and there may be some comfort to be had in that. Now, this is not to say that every critical comment is someone trying to deal with their shit (that would result in us keeping the blinkers on and shutting ourselves off from any ability to self-develop), but it is something worth bearing in mind where criticism is unprovoked and unhelpful.

If you've established that the criticism is helpful, give yourself time to process it. Don't be quick to react. Allow your wellbeing temperature to cool so that when you do respond you are less hot-headed and better able to take on board the suggestions given.

THE 5 SENSE CHALLENGE:
giving it back

While it can be difficult being on the receiving end of criticism, it can sometimes be equally challenging to have to be the 'criticizer'. You may be racked with guilt over how someone has responded. You might feel angry if their defensiveness has resulted in you being left to pick up the pieces of an unfinished job. You might feel upset if offering constructive feedback has left a friendship or relationship hanging by a thread.

How is the feedback you give normally received by others? Does it depend on the individual? How do you feel about giving feedback?

If you find that your experience of giving feedback is a negative one, it may be worth evaluating your approach. A more considered approach can help to make the situation less stressful, protect your and the other individual's mental wellbeing and ensure that you have a positive relationship moving forward.

5 steps to giving feedback:

1. **Timely.** Wherever possible, make sure that you offer the feedback as close to the 'critiquing' situation as possible, rather than allowing ill-feeling to build up. My husband is a pain for leaving dirty laundry on the bedroom floor. Rather than sit and stew about it, I choose to broach the issue with him there and then, as soon as I can.

2. **Stop labelling.** Make sure that when offering criticism, you label the behaviour, not the person. Tempted as I might be to call my husband a slob, it is important that I resist that urge. Rather than label him, I need to label the behaviour and communicate what I don't like about it. '*I wish you would pick up your dirty laundry rather than leaving it on the bedroom floor.*'

3. **Feeling.** Tell them how what they have done has made you feel. '*It's exhausting having to pick up after you.*'

4. **Change.** Communicate what you would like to see change in a calm, clear way. Make sure you are specific. Rather than ask my husband to '*be more considerate*', I need to be clear in what way and make it specific to the situation: '*Could you please make an effort to just pick up your dirty laundry every time you get undressed*.'

5. **Listen and move forward.** Listen to your partner's response and agree what might make it more helpful for them to do this in the future.

Practise these 5 steps next time you are faced with the challenge of having to offer feedback to someone. How did they respond? Did it go better than you anticipated?

Giving feedback is a crucial part of our communication with others, yet is something that a lot of us can still struggle with. Instead, you might find that you hold yourself and your mental wellbeing ransom to the unacceptable behaviour of others. You might jump to conclusions as to what will happen if you give someone feedback.

'*If I tell him to pick up his laundry, he will think I am a nag and he will leave me.*'

'*If I tell her that dress is too tight, she will think I am calling her fat.*'

'*If I tell him that I did the coffee run last week then he will think I am not grateful.*'

Holding back from giving feedback can mean you end up breeding negative or uncomfortable feelings about situations or relationships you find yourself in. You might harbour resentment (which was certainly the case for me every time I was faced with a clothes-ridden floor), guilt (she asked me if she should size up, I should have said yes) or anger (there are 20 other apprentices in the office, why can't they do the coffee run?).

There is a misconception that feedback is *always negative*, but in fact it gives us all opportunity to grow and self-develop. It can also improve communication and trust and enhance your social and working connections.

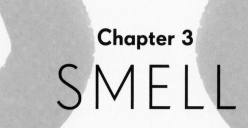

Chapter 3

SMELL

Breathe in: mindfulness and meditation

Early studies suggest that mindfulness and meditation may be helpful in reducing stress, alleviating low mood, aggression and anxiety, and improving quality of life in healthy adults. It has also been found to improve positivity and wellbeing.

Often the terms 'mindfulness' and 'meditation' are used interchangeably, but Headspace. com helpfully explains the subtle differences between the two. Meditation is the skill and experience in developing awareness and compassion, i.e. learning to observe our feelings without judgement for a limited period of time. Meditation is often referred to as the 'training ground for learning mindfulness'.

Mindfulness is then our ability to translate our awareness of the here and now (what we have learned via meditative practice) into our everyday lives; a way of living. This allows us to potentially step back from the chaos of the day, to create moments of being present in the here and now, and to really focus on what we are doing at any given moment or situation. This can be really helpful in allowing us to acknowledge and recognize difficult emotions we may be experiencing and handle these more compassionately.

While there are apps and online programmes that can support mindfulness and meditation, speaking from personal experience I know that exiting an app after a guided meditation may just tempt you to check incoming phone calls, messages, emails and social media notifications. This can be particularly problematic if you are opting to meditate or engage in mindfulness activity before bed.

The exercises I share do not rely on you having to use your devices. They can be done last thing at night and first thing in the morning, or at the end of a working day when you find yourself on a packed tube panicking that others are encroaching on your personal space.

If while practising the exercise overleaf, or my earlier mindfulness exercise, 'the 5 sense countdown' on page 67, you find thoughts entering your mind or you experience unpleasant emotions and feelings, acknowledge these momentarily and then allow yourself to return to the activity. Don't conclude that this means 'it's no good' or it's something that you can't do. Remember, meditative and mindfulness practice is not about ridding your mind of all thought and emotion but about allowing yourself to experience these without judgement.

THE 5 SENSE CHALLENGE:
'pick an object' breathing

Find an object in your eyeline. What shape is it? If it is square/rectangular or even angular (diamond/pentagon/hexagon), follow the edges of the shape on your **breath in** and at each angle point **take a breath out** until you have made your way round the entire shape.

If your shape is more circular or ovoid, focus in on the centre of the shape. Imagine it has been cut into quarters, with an imaginary line from the centre through to the top (the 12 o'clock position), from the centre to the right-hand side (the 3 o'clock position), from the centre to the bottom (the 6 o'clock position) and from the centre to the left-hand side (the 9 o'clock position).

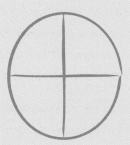

On your breath in, follow the line from the centre to the 12 o'clock position. Hold; then start to breathe out, following the line back down to the centre. On returning to the centre, breathe in, following the line to the 3 o'clock position. Hold; breathe out as you return to the centre.

Now two more to go
On your breath in, follow the line from the centre to the 6 o'clock position.
Hold; then start to breathe out, following the line back up to the centre.
On returning to the centre, breathe in, following the line to the 9 o'clock position.
Hold; breathe out as you return to the centre.

The smell of the great outdoors

Exercise is one of the most undervalued tools for supporting our mental wellbeing. Studies have shown that physical activity can be considered as an evidence-based treatment for depression, with some evidence emerging of its benefit in individuals with anxiety and stress-related disorders. Exercise has also been shown to improve sleep quality as well as reducing sleep latency, i.e. the time it takes for us to fall asleep.

There is also a growing interest and body of evidence developing that looks at the role and importance of 'green exercise' (i.e. exercising in the great outdoors) for our mental wellbeing, with some studies identifying improved self-esteem and mood, particularly with activities done in green spaces close to water.

For many of my patients, regular exercise has helped lift their mood, boost their confidence and improve their self-esteem. For others, it can help them remain focused during the day; to be alert during that early-bird meeting or to be scrupulous when tackling their to-do lists. It can also be a great way to meet other people, to socialize and enhance team building and communication, particularly with group exercise; all essential skills that we do well to bring into our everyday lives.

While we know that exercise has the potential to do all these things, for some of us these benefits often get overlooked in favour of aesthetics, i.e. how exercise makes us *look*.

I know I have been guilty in the past of viewing exercise as a necessity, something I had to do, to earn that calorie-laden snack, or as a means to lose and maintain weight ahead of a holiday. I used to set myself unrealistic expectations around how frequently I should exercise or the number of calories I needed to burn for the workout to be 'worth it' This set up an 'all or nothing' attitude whereby if I didn't meet the targets I'd set myself for any given week or time, I'd conclude that I had come 'off plan' and write off the rest of the exercise or week altogether.

If this sounds all too familiar, often marketing campaigns and group exercises run in military fashion can prey on these vulnerabilities. How familiar does the rhetoric of '*being bad*', '*falling off the wagon*', '*letting yourself go*' or '*needing to punish yourself*' and '*get back on it*' sound to you? I don't know about you, but this terminology can sometimes have the opposite effect to its motivational intention. Exercise then becomes something to fear, to dread, a tool to punish and fundamentally not enjoy.

I am happy to say that in the last ten years my attitude to exercise has completely changed. My life has got a lot busier, so logistically fitting it in has been more difficult with juggling the demands of a busy job, becoming a wife and mum. I have redefined for myself what constitutes exercise, weakening the torturous black-and-white thinking of either going to the gym all the time or not bothering with exercise at all. While in my 20s I would have only considered a workout to count if it was done at the gym, I now view a run around the park with my daughter or parking my car in the furthest bay and getting some extra steps in to be just as valid.

I am also clear on the reasons why I exercise. As I've got older, and with impressionable ears and eyes in the shape of my 5-year-old around, I am moving away from exercising for the reasons other people or objects tell me to (extrinsic reasons) and am focusing more on exercising because of how it makes me feel (intrinsic) – happier and more energized.

If you only view exercise from the narrow focal point of what you stand to lose (namely weight), you shut yourself off from what you stand to *gain* from it.

Ask yourself

Do you exercise?

....

....

....

How often?

....

....

....

What does your exercise look like?
Walking to/from work? Running in the great outdoors? Swimming? Going to the gym x times a week?

....

....

....

What are the reasons you exercise?

....

....

....

THE 5 SENSE CHALLENGE:
exercise log

Record your exercise for a typical week using the log below. This can be anything from deciding to take the stairs instead of the lift, to your weekly spin or daily yoga flow. State when the exercise took place, the type of exercise and the reason why you have done it.

Record your wellbeing temperature before and after you work out.

Do you track your activity? If so, why?
Is it for health reasons, curiosity or is it a means of holding yourself accountable?

....

....

....

Use the notes section to jot down any thoughts that come to mind after the exercise has been completed.

'I'm so annoyed I didn't push myself as hard as I hoped.'

Or:

'I haven't earned that cupcake.'

Day	Type of Exercise	Reason	Before	After	Track? Y/N	Notes

How did you get on? Does your log surprise you? What proportion of your exercises do you do for your mental or physical health, and what is done purely because you feel *you have to*, as a means of punishment or to 'earn' something?

By being aware of how and why we exercise, we can make choices that benefit us rather than make us feel more pressure to look a certain way.

Ask yourself

In much the same way that we have spoken about the need to clear out negative friendships or tasks that don't serve us, it is time to exercise (excuse the pun) the same level of scrutiny on our workouts. For the exercises that you have highlighted as doing purely as a means of punishment, run through the following screening questions:

Do I *truly enjoy* the exercise? YES/NO

If doing it meant that I *wouldn't* lose weight or burn x amount of calories, would I still do it? YES/NO

These might feel like difficult questions to answer, but are important to address all the same. If you want to develop a positive relationship with exercise that you can sustain in the long term, making the distinction between it being something that you inflict on yourself for extrinsic reasons at the expense of the intrinsic, and how it makes you feel, is an important one to make.

If you view all your exercise as a means of punishment, consider what exercise, given the option, you would like to do instead. These exercises may well be things you have written off previously, for instance '*because you don't think that they will burn enough calories*'.

....

....

....

Our need for external validation remains a common theme within this book, and rightly so. If it is something you fall foul of, it is important to understand the power you give to others to determine how you feel about yourself and your self-esteem, and start to regain that control for yourself. We've all been there. You might have worked super hard during a workout class and feel really proud for pushing yourself, only to turn to your tracker and feel deflated by the number that suggests otherwise. Tracking can also set up unhealthy 'trade-off' relationships between exercise and food: '*If I eat this I can work it off later*' or '*If I work out now then I can pig out later*'.

THE 5 SENSE CHALLENGE:
the exercise contract

Switching it up. Each week, aim to replace one punishing exercise with an enjoyable exercise.

Think about the gains. Remind yourself of what you stand to gain from doing the exercise – being more focused, happier and getting a better night's sleep.

What positives do you personally notice after exercise?

....

....

....

Stop tracking. It's unbelievable the responsibility we place on others or on objects (fitness trackers, calorie burn on a piece of equipment) to dictate how we should be feeling before, during or after a workout.

Not burned enough calories? We feel inadequate, low or anxious.

Calorie burn on point? We are elated and feel 'in control'.

Smelling the bullshit

We have already discussed the impact that social media use in general can have on your mental wellbeing. Were it not enough that you have access to vast amounts of information at your fingertips, you have the added challenge of needing to vet out the unreliable and potentially damaging information you come into contact with – the bullshit. This bullshit can sometimes lead you to question aspects of your own life and set up feelings of indadequacy. Being confronted with the latest quick-fix fat-loss cure may lead you to doubt your 'slow' efforts of eating well and exercising regularly. Being presented with someone's constant posts of adoration for their partner may force you to dwell on an argument you had with your own earlier in the day and instil doubt about the closeness of your relationship.

Have the courage to be more critical. Are you quick to shut down cold callers trying to sell you something that doesn't quite add up? If so, what stops you practising the same level of scrutiny in other areas of your life? Think about what you might do in the case of the cold caller. You may initially politely decline the offer made. If they persist or continue to push you with their commission in tow, you might be more abrupt in your defence and tell them where to stick it.

Meet Antonia:

Another Monday morning had rolled around, and Antonia had declared that she was going to sign up to the latest celebrity weight-loss shake programme. 'This is it', she declared to her shared office. 'This is the plan that is going to get me down to a size 8. All I have to do is just drink three of these shakes a day for the next four weeks.

'If it's good enough for [insert chosen celebrity] then it's good enough for me.'

We reflected on how Antonia might react if she heard one of her friends embarking on a similar mission. She admitted that she would probably be more than a little sceptical. She agreed that it was a lot of money to part with, but concluded that she had no choice. In her own words, she was 'lazy and lacked willpower'. We reflected on why she held this opinion of herself, and it became apparent that she was starting to adopt some of the brand's marketing speak.

'Why do you think they might be telling you that you have no willpower?'

'To get me to buy their shakes.'

The penny dropped.

I wondered if Antonia's readiness to buy into something was translatable to all areas of life. I asked her, 'If you didn't drive and I told you that you needed a car, would you buy one from me?' She confidently answered that she wouldn't.

'What if you did drive and I told you that you should only buy a car from me?' Caveat: I have no experience with cars. Antonia concluded that she wouldn't buy one from me due to my lack of experience and would more than likely go to a car dealer.

We reflected on two issues here, the first being that we are drawn in by the promise of what someone or something can do for us, and the second being that we are willing to compromise our health and turn a blind eye to expertise in the process if the 'profile' is big enough. Antonia was able to accept that this celebrity objectively had very few credentials when it came to selling this product, but the 'it worked for her, therefore it will work for me' testimonial was all the proof she needed.

Conversely, Antonia was able to confidently turn down my attempts to sell her something on the basis that I didn't have any experience. But why should two people with a similar objective (trying to sell Antonia something) produce completely different outcomes?

Why is it that on the one hand Antonia is able to protect herself (by ensuring that she gets advice from a car dealer who is reputable) but on the other compromises her health and bank balance to commit to a diet shake programme from someone unqualified?

Meet Alison:

Alison is preparing for her university finals. She is stressing out about the volume of work she has to cover. She sets about organizing a revision timetable that she diligently sticks to. She splits her time between revising at home, setting up residence at the local coffee shop, and late-evening sessions at the university library. During one of her library sessions, her friend Karen sidles up to her with no revision material in sight. Karen shares that she has 'literally done no work and is totally going to flunk it'.

Alison goes on to pass the exam, while Karen manages to pass with honours.

Alison inevitably found herself drawing comparisons between herself and Karen. She can't fathom why she has to work harder than Karen to 'just scrape by'.

We reflected on whether anyone could get as good a result as Karen without putting the work in. Alison was able to acknowledge that a complete novice probably couldn't. Which begged the question, why bullshit?

Why do we bullshit?

Reflecting on both the digital and IRL examples on the previous pages, the common theme that we see and hear about is this idea that the person selling us something (a product, an idea or a belief) is 100% correct because '*they have said so*'. Fundamentally, someone who is bullshitting you is trying to sell you something for their own gain. In this digital age of influencer marketing, the transparency of paid partnerships and #spon makes the gain clear – your money. If it's not monetary, it is to sell you a belief or an ideal.

Bullshitting in real life, as in Karen's case, may be due to several factors. It may reflect Karen's own insecurities. Karen may have in fact put the hours of revision in but may be in self-preservation mode, so if she does fluff up, then '*it's OK because she had others believe she didn't put the work in anyway*'.

Conversely, Karen might be bullshitting because she wants others to believe that she is 'effortlessly bright' and 'that it comes naturally to her'; the ego-massage.

Whatever Karen's reasons for bullshitting, it leads Alison to draw comparisons with herself based *only* on what Karen has *chosen* to share: the false truth, i.e. that she is doing next to no revision but yet still manages to come out on top.

It is also important to bear in mind that bullshit might be a tactic used to spare your feelings. Ever asked a friend how your hair looked after some dodgy hairdresser has been at it? Yes, me too. In this situation, while there might be a mutual understanding that some bullshit is being spread, the '*it's fine, honestly*', both parties agree that it is helpful and not harmful; the friend who doesn't want to upset a friend (the bullshitter) and the bullshittee wanting the peace of mind that they look 'OK' even if they know they don't.

THE 5 SENSE CHALLENGE:
smelling the bullshit detector

Next time you find yourself on the receiving end of bullshit, run through the following checklist to help you approach the situation more critically. By becoming wise to when someone is bullshitting and reflecting on the reasons why they might be doing so, you can protect yourself from the negative impact it may otherwise have had.

- **Who** is the bullshitter?
- **What** are they telling you?
- **Why** are they telling you?
- Do they have the experience to sell you this? This is particularly relevant for those 'too good to be true' products or plans.
- Does your instinct tell you it is too good to be true?
- How does their possible bullshit make you **feel**?
- How does their bullshit make you **act**?
- Is their bullshitting an annoyance or is it harmful (affecting you physically or emotionally or both)?

If the bullshit detector leads you to conclude that you are dealing with bullshit, do not buy into the idea, belief or product. Politely decline, mute or walk away, depending on how the bullshit has presented itself. Tell yourself that it is bullshit and remind yourself of the reasons why an individual or product might be telling you this. Remind yourself of the negative impact that buying into the bullshit will have on you.

Sweet smell of success

Throughout your lifetime, you may set yourself a number of life goals that you wish to achieve. Some of these goals you may be able to achieve with relatively little difficulty, whereas others may feel further out of reach, with possibly fear even holding you back from attaining them. You might feel frustrated by your inability to be more expressive with what you wear for fear that you can't pull it off. You might feel helpless about remaining in your 9 to 5 but fear you are not quite good enough for anything else.

The longer you put off tackling your goals, the more reinforced the idea that they are 'unattainable' or 'out of reach' will become...

Ask yourself

What personal, professional or social goals would you like to achieve in life? Jot your goals down at the top of the hill.

....

....

....

How far out of reach do these goals feel for you at the moment?

Where are you *on that hill at the moment? The bottom of the hill is not even close and the top of the hill is achieving your goals. Mark this point with an x.*

How **specific** are your goals?

Is there a way of demonstrating when you have reached these goals? Often patients I see may decide they '*want to be more confident*'. While this is an admirable goal, because it is so general it is quite difficult to tangibly measure and to truly establish when it has been achieved.

However, a goal of being more confident by being able to '*wear something that you wouldn't have otherwise*' is something that is more tangible, and one you can demonstrate that you have or haven't achieved relatively easily.

THE 5 SENSE CHALLENGE:
planning your trek

Using the hill opposite, **define** your goal and plan your own trek to success.

Remind yourself of **why** you want to achieve this goal. Stick this hill somewhere that is clearly visible. During the trek, which may take several weeks, months or years in some cases, you may lose sight of why this goal is important to you.

Make a plan. Think about what experience you already have. What do you need to do? By when? What other tools do you need to help you on your way?

Set yourself mini-goals en route. It is important to celebrate when you achieve each of these. These will help keep you on track, boost your confidence and motivate you during moments of self-doubt.

Imagine deciding to climb Mount Everest – you would rarely do this without sufficient preparation. You would decide what you needed to do, by when, and determine what you needed to bring with you.

You might already have some experience of trekking that puts you in good stead.

You may well have mapped out your route and planned ahead for possible obstacles that come your way.

You might decide to set yourself a series of practice treks (mini-treks) to build up your stamina, increase your confidence and your motivation to tackle your ultimate goal.

All these steps ensure that you are successful in your mission to climb Mount Everest. The goals that you set yourself in life should be no different.

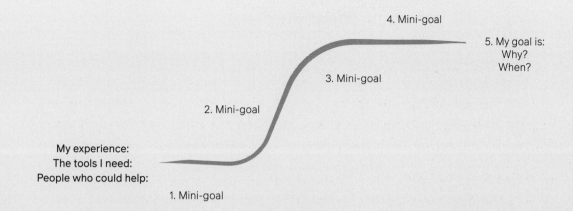

4. Mini-goal

5. My goal is:
Why?
When?

3. Mini-goal

2. Mini-goal

My experience:
The tools I need:
People who could help:

1. Mini-goal

Notes

....

....

....

....

....

....

Meet Andrew:

Andrew has just moved to a new city. He is in a flatshare with a couple of professionals he has only just met. Each week, they make an effort to sit down and have dinner together. Andrew is struggling to find his voice, particularly as the others are both big personalities. He wishes he could be more confident, particularly during their weekly catch-up, in offering his opinions rather than sitting in silence and taking it in.

Andrew defines his specific goal and we think about the mini-goals that might help to make reaching it more achievable.

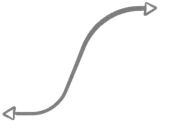

My goal is:
speaking out during weekly flatshare dinners

Why?
So my opinion is heard and I can build relationships

When?
Within the next couple of months

My experience:
all my friendships started from somewhere

The tools I need:
self-confidence, learning to use my voice

People that could help:
friends, work colleagues I trust

Mini-goal 1	Mini-goal 2	Mini-goal 3	Mini-goal 4	Specific goal
Giving an opinion while out with a close friend	Non-verbally (nodding/shaking head) agreeing/disagreeing with banter	Verbally asking for something during the meal	Contributing to the weekly banter by commenting on the topic being spoken about	Starting own topic of conversation in the weekly banter

Getting yourself from the bottom of the hill to the top

Being faced with your ultimate goal from the off can feel overwhelming and unsafe – expecting Andrew to take the lead in conversation with his flatmates, for instance, will only set him up to fail. He will more than likely feel overwhelmed with anxiety and convince himself that he is not able to do it, and may abandon the trek (goal) altogether.

It is important that each of the mini-goals you set yourself still makes you feel a little anxious (red or orange), not quite as much as your ultimate goal but certainly enough to challenge you. Each goal should gradually become more difficult and bring you one step closer to your ultimate goal. Avoid setting the bar too high, particularly for your first mini-goal. Struggling to get beyond the first hurdle may just compound how unachievable you believe the final goal to be – 'I can't do it', 'I am always going to struggle with this' – while having at least one achievement under your belt mentally can be incredibly encouraging and motivate you to tackle the next.

Before trekking up to the next mini-goal, ensure you repeat each goal until your wellbeing temperature comes down to a blue or green.

This allows you to habituate to the anxiety such that over time and through repeated exposure, the negative impact it has on you weakens.

The Goal Review

Review your goals each week:

How does tackling that mini-goal now make you feel?

....

....

....

How many times have you attempted to tackle it this week?

....

....

....

If you are still rating your wellbeing temperature as a red, reflect on the challenges you faced.

....

....

....

What do you think you need to bear in mind for the following week to help you achieve this mini-goal and move on to the next?

....

....

....

Are your goals realistic? Do you need to break them down into even simpler ones?

....

....

....

Make a commitment to attempt your goal again.

Suggest a date and time to repeat your mini-goal or goal.

Make sure that it is **within the next 7 days so that you have opportunity to review your progress weekly**.

Remember, the longer you put off tackling your goals, the more reinforced the idea that they are 'unattainable' or 'out of reach' will become and the longer you will continue to avoid or fear them.

Don't jump ahead or 'miss out' mini-goals altogether, even if you feel confident to do so. Remember when you were a child and would jump every couple of steps just to clear the staircase more quickly? If you were anything like me, you were probably scolded – *be careful or you'll fall*. It's the same principle: jump steps too quickly and you are likely to fall, which may make you less confident about re-attempting them. Take your time and you are more likely to clear the staircase safely and reach the top.

THE 5 SENSE CHALLENGE:
the dreaded to-do list

If you are anything like me, you can often feel overwhelmed by an ever-growing to-do list in which things seemingly never get done. Rather than invest what valuable time you do have in completing the tasks, you instead find yourself procrastinating or worrying that you won't ever get around to completing them. Another day, another week rolls around and you are no further forwards. In the meantime, you continue to amass more and more things that *need doing*, putting you under increasing strain. So, how do you make your to-do lists more functional and in turn ease the pressure you may be under?

At the start of each week, write down a list of the **things that you need to do**.

Beside each item on the list, write down the deadline for **when** this needs to be done by.

Why does it need to be completed by then? For instance, if I don't pay this bill by [insert date] then I will get a fine.

Rank your list depending on deadlines, where the top (RED) are the things that need to be done as soon as possible and the bottom are the things that can wait and don't necessarily have a deadline (BLUE) and transfer the list to the table opposite.

Specify **how long** you need for each task and **what day** you will set aside time to do this. You might find that if a certain item is ongoing, such as writing a dissertation, you might diarize this in every day but limit yourself to half a day at any one time.

Avoid overfilling any one day with all your red and orange tasks – try to spread these throughout the week if deadlines will allow.

When you only focus on the things you know you **need** to get done but more often than not are the most time-consuming or complex (RED), you may feel frustrated that you are not getting them done quickly enough. You may procrastinate because they struggle to hold your attention for long enough; you reach a saturation point. This may mean that you never get around to clearing those simpler tasks that are not likely to be as taxing or take quite so long, but nonetheless contribute to the overall load.

Do not give yourself any more than 5 to-dos to tackle in any given day.

Each morning draw up your to-do list of 5 items for that day.

Put it somewhere you can see it.

At the end of the day tick off which tasks you have managed to complete.

Are there any that you did not complete that you need to roll on to another day? Look back at your week's schedule, is there any room to fit this into the remainder of the week, or if deadlines will allow can this be postponed to the following week?

To do	How long	Day	Completed by

Continues overleaf

To do	How long	Day	Completed by

Scents, sleep and all things self-care

You've probably all heard the term 'self-care' thrown around, but what does it actually mean and what constitutes good self-care? There is no one right way to self-care. Self-care for me might look very different from self-care for you. Either way, self-care is what you do yourself *purposefully* to look after your mental and physical wellbeing. It can constitute anything from mindfulness and exercise, which we have covered in the previous two sections, to burning a candle, running a bath, baking or being outdoors.

If your life only ever seems to be getting busier, it's all too easy to forget to take time out for yourself. If you are anything like me, when you do eventually stop for a minute to do something for yourself you feel an immense rush of guilt. You push yourself further and further down the priority list.

Self-care isn't and shouldn't be complicated. The majority of what you have read so far within this book constitutes self-care, from the social media curfew, to listening to your internal 'no', to exercising. Rather than self-care being an afterthought, something you do only once everyone and everything is taken care of and only then if you have time, it should be something you do as a matter of routine. In much the same way that you would book an appointment or meeting, you should make a concerted effort to book an appointment with yourself. Physically booking an appointment sets up that accountability – '*It's in the diary, therefore I have to commit to it*' – rather than it being a hypothetical thing that you never get around to doing or that other things get prioritized over instead.

Each day, ensure you set aside some time to practise self-care.

It can be:

- Lighting a candle while you read uninterrupted, for half an hour each evening.
- An indulgent evening bath every day/week.
- A phone-free lunch break or escaping from your desk.

The key is it has to be something that you book in and commit to each day. Aim for at least 30 minutes of self-care a day.

You may find it easier to plan your self-care at the start of each day. Or it may be more convenient for you to plan ahead and schedule self-care appointments for the week ahead on a Sunday evening. Either way, it is essential you put pen to paper or create an e-appointment with yourself, using your phone, tablet or laptop to set up that accountability and ensure it is something that you 'attend'.

Ask yourself

Think about what things you do that come under the umbrella of self-care.

....

....

....

Do you regularly book in appointments with yourself?

....

....

....

How strictly do you keep to these appointments? Do you fit in self-care whenever you can, or is it something that you commit to regularly; daily/weekly?

....

....

....

THE 5 SENSE CHALLENGE:
self-care roulette

If you are stuck for self-care ideas, self-care roulette is a great tool to use to spark inspiration. Grab a piece of paper and write down each of the self-care activities below. Tear each idea off, then fold them up and throw them into a bowl or empty jam jar. Each day pick out a self-care activity at random to complete. Feel free to add other activities to the self-care roulette list below that might better reflect your interests.

Prefer to plan for the week ahead? Pick out 7 activities each Sunday evening and schedule these into your diary at the start of each week.

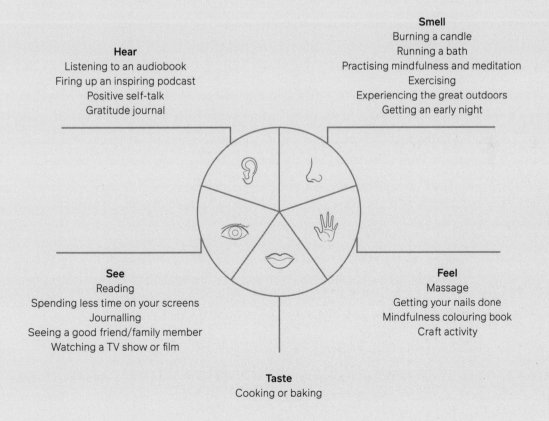

Smell
Burning a candle
Running a bath
Practising mindfulness and meditation
Exercising
Experiencing the great outdoors
Getting an early night

Hear
Listening to an audiobook
Firing up an inspiring podcast
Positive self-talk
Gratitude journal

See
Reading
Spending less time on your screens
Journalling
Seeing a good friend/family member
Watching a TV show or film

Feel
Massage
Getting your nails done
Mindfulness colouring book
Craft activity

Taste
Cooking or baking

Sleep as self-care

Daily, I see patients in clinic who struggle with their sleep. Usually, their problem is difficulty getting to sleep, staying asleep or waking up too early, if not a combination. One of the things I like to do is unpack what their evening routine looks like. This helps me think about some of the barriers that might make getting to sleep more difficult. Unsurprisingly, for many of them a screen isn't far from reach, and in some cases they might be guilty of 'multi-screen multi-tasking'. Ever find yourself simultaneously scrolling through your phone, sending a text to a friend, watching Netflix in the background and maybe even working on a project on your laptop at the same time? That's an awful lot of stimulation for one day, let alone one evening!

Your evening routine should be about unwinding and prepping your mind and body for sleep, particularly those crucial couple of hours before lights out. Yet we do everything in our power (binge-watching box sets, the mindless scroll) to sabotage that, keeping ourselves awake in the process. If you struggle to log off in the evening, you end up over-stimulating your mind at a time when it should be slowing down, so it is little wonder that your brain never quite gets the cue to switch off.

When we hear about screen use in the evening, the perils of blue light are never far away! Exposure to blue light in the evening suppresses melatonin – a crucial hormone that helps regulate our sleep and wake cycles, and that relies on darkness in order to be produced. The blue light tricks our bodies into thinking that it is still daytime (or light), so our pineal gland (the gland in our brain that produces the melatonin) never gets the cue that it is night-time and that it needs to start producing melatonin to prepare us for sleep.

In short, disrupted sleep/wake cycles can affect both the quantity and quality of our sleep, which not only spells disaster the following day (struggling to concentrate, poor performance, lack of energy) but can also wreak havoc on our physical and mental health in the long term. Loss of sleep has been linked to heart disease, weight gain, obesity and diabetes, and has even been shown to affect our reproductive and immune systems.

What should you be doing with your screens in the evening? Does a perfect evening routine exist? Is there a one-size-fits-all approach?

If you are struggling with your sleep and are a slave to your screen in the evening, it may be worth putting some limits in place. In much the same way that I suggest a morning screen curfew, an evening screen curfew can be equally helpful. It also helps to set up clear distinctions between your day and night, your work and downtime. What is making the latter increasingly more difficult, however, is how much our working lives have changed over the years. You may be juggling more than one job. You may be working shifts. Your working day may no longer start the minute your bum hits the seat in an office or end the moment you clock off at 5. I know I am guilty of heavily blurring the boundaries on my commute to and from work, taking calls and checking and responding to emails.

In addition to looking at screen use, I help my patients identify other barriers to a good night using the 5 sense framework below.

SEE

- **Screens**. Are you using screened devices right up to going to bed? Many of my patients were reading books using e-readers or iPads and still struggling to go to sleep. Studies have shown that individuals reading from an e-reader compared with a printed book took longer to fall asleep. E-reading before bed suppresses the release of melatonin by as much as 50% compared to a printed book. This impacts the quality of your sleep and your alertness the following day.

- **Exposure to light**. Your brain, more specifically the suprachiasmatic nucleus (your 24-hour body clock), relies on the repeated pattern of loss of light (night) and return of light (day) to help reset it. Commuting to and from work in the dark, limited daylight exposure in the day (think high-rise windowless office blocks), and the use of artificial, bright lights in the evening can upset your 24-hour body clock.

HEAR

- **Loud environment**. I know only too well the impact that a loud environment can have on sleep. My daughter was a colicky baby, which often meant hours of desperately trying to settle her right up until midnight. But while she passed out from exhausting herself with all that crying, I found myself buzzing and wide awake. Noisy neighbours, living on a busy road and snoring partners can also mean that your sleeping environment is less than desirable.

- **Not listening to your internal cues**. The nights out you insist on going on when you could do with an early night, the heavy eyelids and constant yawning when you are three episodes deep into a thrilling box set – your body is pretty adept at communicating when it is ready for bed, yet you might choose to ignore these cues.

SMELL

- **Exercising too late** in the evening can make the onset of sleep more difficult. This is thought to be related to the increase in metabolic rate and subsequent rise in core body temperature following exercise. As well as loss of light, drop of body temperature is also needed to initiate sleep.

- **Passing on mindfulness and meditation strategies**. Constantly being on the go and having to 'do, do, do'.

FEEL

- **Are you comfortable**? You would be surprised how important your immediate sleeping environment is for getting a good night. Uncomfortable mattress, thin bedding, too hot or too cold bedroom – all these factors can impact how quickly you get to sleep and how restful the sleep is.

- **Feeling worried**. A lot of the patients I see are consumed by worry right before going to bed, ruminating over the things they have done that day, the future and the things that might not ever happen. Before they know it, it is the other side of midnight.

TASTE

- **Caffeine too late at night**. Are you partial to an afternoon coffee or an evening cuppa before bed? And don't forget the hidden caffeine in colas, energy drinks, protein supplements and chocolate. Caffeine is a stimulant. It makes you more alert – not synonymous with the unwind before bed. It can take up to 7 hours for just half the caffeine in your evening cuppa to work its way out of your system.

- **Alcohol**. You might be partial to a glass of wine after work, or a cheeky nightcap, but alcohol's sedative effects mean that it only initiates a lighter, superficial sleep. It can also result in restlessness and wakefulness in the night.

THE 5 SENSE CHALLENGE:
cleaning up your sleep routine

To optimize your sleep, try cleaning up your sleep routine.

Create a schedule and stick to it. Go to bed at the same time each night and wake up at the same time each morning, even on a weekend. This helps regulate your 24-hour clock or circadian rhythm.

Avoid using screened devices 1–2 hours before bed. That includes everything from phones, to tablets, laptops and TVs. Keep all screens and devices out of the bedroom. Wherever possible, charge phones elsewhere and invest in a good old-fashioned alarm clock. If you are likely to forget about your screen curfew, set an alarm 1–2 hours before you are due to go to bed, to remind yourself that it is time to switch off.

If the lure of a device is too tempting, ensure that you turn off your notifications and switch to airplane mode.

Read books in print.

Invest in a blackout blind for your bedroom, particularly in those pesky summer months.

Get exposure to natural daylight in the day. If you are commuting to and from work in the dark, use your lunch break or lunch hour to leave your desk and go for a walk outside.

Invest in some ear plugs and soundproof your bedroom.

Listen to your body's signals that you are tired (yawning, heavy eyelids) and take yourself off to bed.

Practise mindfulness and meditation. Practise one of the exercises in 'Breathe in: mindfulness and meditation' (page 111) each evening before bed.

Avoid exercising too late at night, preferably no later than at least 2–3 hours before bed.

Run yourself a bath before bed. The drop in body temperature afterwards can make you feel sleepier.

Keep a worry journal by your bed to 'dump' your worries into. More on 'worry dumps' and 'worry curfews' on page 150.

Avoid caffeinated drinks in the afternoon and evening.

Avoid consuming alcohol.

Evening screen curfew

If you absolutely can't avoid screen use in the evening, you might want to consider some of the blue-light blocking devices or filters which appear to have exploded in popularity recently, from apps that can be downloaded on to your phone to the glasses that you can wear while navigating your screens. Personally, this is not something that I have ever recommended to the patients I see, and hence I won't be making any specific product recommendations here. The reason being that while some of these products may be shown to block blue light frequency, I still believe that it is the activity itself (the working on an assignment late at night, scrolling the internet mindlessly or the emotional messages to/from a friend) that has just as significant an impact, if not more, on our wakefulness, due to the emotions it stirs up within us that may make getting to sleep more difficult.

When I suggest an evening screen curfew, I am often met with confusion or horror that there lies an existence beyond our phones. So, what other activities might you choose to do instead?

Screen-free alternatives in the evening:

Read. Curl up with a good book, magazine or journal.

Journal. You may have made steps to change certain unhelpful behaviours as part of your 5 senses plan. Use this as an opportunity to reflect on how far you have come and how much closer you are to achieving the goal(s) you have set yourself.

Preparation. Avoid that dash first thing on a morning and use the slumber hour to lay out your clothes, pack your bag or prepare your breakfast or lunch for the following day.

Gratitude. Feeling grateful? We know that gratitude exercises can harness positivity and may help us to refocus and take stock of objects, attributes and relationships that are meaningful and valuable to us; the good in our lives. Studies have shown that gratitude can make us more optimistic and more likely to behave in ways that maintain a healthy lifestyle. Improved sleep, better self-esteem and mood are just a few of the positives we stand to gain from practising gratitude regularly. Invest in a notepad or diary and jot down three things that you are grateful for at the end of each day. You may want to make it a communal affair and it might be an activity that you do with a partner or a close friend.

Worry dump. Feeling anxious or on edge before bed? Then put your worries to paper (and to bed – excuse the pun). For more information on this, jump ahead to 'Time to worry' (page 147).

Mindfulness. For mindfulness tools and techniques, look back at 'Breathe in: mindfulness and meditation' (page 111).

Sex. Time spent with a loved one can often be sacrificed to a device or three. We prioritize digital connections over our physical, more tangible ones. Use your screen curfew time as an opportunity to reconnect.

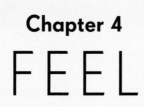

Chapter 4

FEEL

Time to worry

Solutions, not problems

If there is one emotion that I feel dominates all emotions for me, it is worry. I worry constantly. I worry from the moment I wake up right through to the moment I go to sleep. I worry about getting my daughter and myself to school and work respectively on time. I worry about my patients. I worry about my family. I worry about money. I worry about trying to do it all – be a good mum, a wife, a daughter, a sister, an auntie, a friend and an employee. I worry about what people think of me. I worry about illness and death.

Some of these worries can be all-consuming at times. They might see me push myself to the edge and risk burnout. They might lead me to procrastinate over what I ought to be doing, which only serves to make me worry more that I won't get whatever it is done in time. Some of these worries I can do something about, but other worries might not even happen and so are difficult to prepare for or problem-solve.

It Might Never Happen

Problem-solving worry (PS)

Worry can serve a purpose – for instance, if you are worried that you might flunk an interview or an audition, it might force you to prepare for it. Here you can recognize the worry as a valid problem that you can solve, i.e. instead of worrying about it, you can prepare or practise your routine to make sure that you get the job or part.

'Might not' worry (MN)

In some situations, the problem that's worrying you can't be identified quite so easily, and therefore cannot be easily solved.

For example, what if you're worried that on the way to the interview you get knocked down by a car, break your leg and never make it to the interview, which means you're jobless for ever? You might spend valuable prep time worrying about this one thing that 'might not' even happen. You end up self-fulfilling the prophecy (that you are not going to get the job) because instead of using your time productively you are distracted by worry. Unlike the PS worry, you are unable to turn the MN worry into something solvable – how do you prepare yourself for something that might not even happen?

Worry can serve a purpose – for instance, if you are worried that you might flunk an interview or an audition, it might force you to prepare for it.

Meet Zoe:

Zoe fancied trying a new gym class one evening. Not managing to rope in any of her friends to join her, she decided to go all the same. She worried first about running late (PS worry) and second that she wouldn't know any of the moves and would end up making a fool of herself (MN worry). Zoe spent so long 'might not' worrying about embarrassing herself that she almost ran late for her class as a result, self-fulfilling her other worry. I spoke to Zoe about her worries. We conceded that her worry about being late could be legitimate but that it was something that could be solved relatively easily, i.e. preparing herself to minimize the chances of being late, such as setting herself an alarm, setting off early, etc. Zoe was able to recognize that the time spent worrying about embarrassing herself in the class was redundant. She couldn't do anything there and then about something that might not even happen.

Zoe agreed to setting herself a worry curfew every evening 6–6.30 p.m., as she was waiting for her dinner to cook. When she faced a 'might not' worry before this time, she would instead say out loud, 'This is a "might not" worry, I will think about this later on during my curfew.' She would quickly jot down what the worry was on the notes section on her phone, and move on from it and come back to it during her curfew.

If the worry was a problem-solving worry, then she would turn it into a problem and work out how to solve it using the problem-solving tool – the WWH method (detailed on page 152).

By the time her curfew rolled around, she realized her worry hadn't happened and she didn't need to spend time worrying about it.

THE 5 SENSE CHALLENGE:
worry curfew

I developed the worry curfew as a way of giving my patients permission to worry but allowing them to be in control of *when* they do it, to avoid it causing too much disruption to their day. The worry curfew is about giving yourself a set window in the day during which you can do your 'might not' worrying.

When you catch yourself worrying in the day, ask yourself: 'Is this something that I can do anything about right now, i.e. a problem-solving worry?' If it isn't, then say out loud (or quietly to yourself if you would rather): '*This is a "might not" worry. I'm not going to worry about it now, but I will save it for my curfew later on in the day*.' Quickly jot the worry down in the notes section of your phone or in a journal to come back to during your curfew.

Even if you find the same worry popping into your mind throughout the day, repeat the process. Briefly acknowledge it, jot it down and come back to it later. While it may seem repetitive, it will help reinforce the pattern that 'might not' worries need to be postponed to your curfew.

Similarly, if you find yourself worrying most in the evening, to the extent that it is impacting your sleep, temporarily park these worries, jot them down in your journal and come back to them during your worry curfew.

During your worry curfew:

Review your list of worries. You now have permission to worry freely about these for the next [insert minutes allocated].

Strike out anything no longer worrying you. Jot down what continuing to have worried about this during the day might have done, e.g. *could have wasted time, could have fallen behind with work*.

Classify each worry as either a problem-solving or a 'might not' worry. For the most part, the worries you jot down for your curfew will be 'might not' worries, but if you have had some late-night worrying that is affecting your ability to sleep, you may temporarily park a problem-solving worry until the morning, when you can look at it and identify a solution.

If it's a problem-solving worry, use the problem-solving tool detailed overleaf (the WWH method) to help identify a solution.

Record your wellbeing temperature; where red is an all-consuming worry and blue is 'it is no longer a worry for me'.

Use the tent analogy from page 50 to think about what evidence you have that this worry is or isn't going to happen. How will continuing to worry about this worry serve you?

Once your worry time is complete, tear off the paper from your journal, screw it up and throw it away. Or if you are going digital, delete the note from the notes section of your phone and from your archive. Start afresh the following day.

Practice makes perfect. You may find that the first few times you try this exercise you feel a little awkward, just worrying about worrying for a finite period of time each day; but what you will notice is that you will worry less frequently during the day because of the understanding that you have '*time to do it later*'. You may also become more productive during the day because you are able to identify the worries that can be turned into problems and actioned immediately. And for those 'might not' worries, by the time 'later' rolls around, some of those worries may no longer be of relevance to you and may even be struck off your list.

THE 5 SENSE CHALLENGE:
the WWH method

I developed the WWH (what, who, how) method as a way of helping people work through their worries and try to find a potential solution.

Using the chart below, work through the following steps:

Define your worry: my worry is . . . ?

What support do you need to stop worrying about this?

Who might be able to help?

How might I go about solving this worry?

and

List all the possible solutions for this worry, including the **pros and cons for each. Rank them** in order of which solution sounds the most preferable, tackling each solution in turn until the problem is solved.

For example, Zoe's problem-solving tool might look a little like this:

Define	What	Who	How	Pros	Cons	Rank
Going to be late for workout class	Car	Myself	Drive	Can be in charge of my own timings	May be traffic, have to worry about parking	3
Going to be late for workout class	Tube	Tube driver, fiancé	Walk to tube station or get fiancé to give me lift	Have a couple of people helping me, avoid traffic, don't need to worry about parking	Tube delays, strikes	2
Going to be late for workout class	Taxi	Taxi driver	Ring taxi company	Someone else driving, don't have to worry about parking	Costs money, may be traffic	1

Outcome: having considered all her options, Zoe decides that getting a taxi to her workout will be most preferable because it saves her having to worry about parking and she can predetermine what time to set off.

WWH problem-solving tool

Have a go at completing your own problem-solving tool.

Define		What	Who	How	Pros	Cons	Rank

Perfectly imperfect

Ever place expectation on yourself '*to be perfect*', without flaw? If you do, you might set yourself high standards. You live by what I like to call the 'I must, otherwise I am' rule.

I must not make a mistake, otherwise people will think I am useless.
I must eat clean, otherwise I am or will get fat.
I must not cry, otherwise I am weak.
I must not slip up during that conversation, otherwise I am boring.

While there is nothing wrong with striving to be better and do better, it is important to be realistic about the expectations you place on yourself to get from A (where you are) to B (where you want to be). There is an idea that your journey through life needs to be smooth and free from error if it is to be valid. Any setback can be seen as a failure rather than an opportunity to grow. Speak to any successful individual, entrepreneur, athlete or influencer – what did their journey to success look like? Path A or Path B?

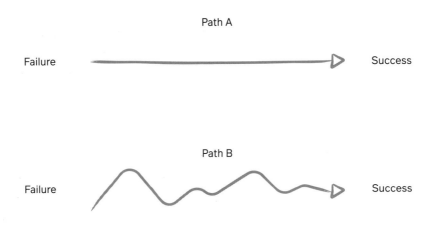

Guaranteed more often than not, their path looked more like Path B, in that they had a few 'less than perfect' slip-ups en route but were able to achieve their end goal nonetheless. However, we convince ourselves that the finished product (them being successful, being the top of their game, hitting a personal best or having x amount of followers) came easily to them, free from error, and followed a perfect path. Unless you live and breathe every minute of every day in someone else's shoes, you can never be 100% sure which path their journey truly resembles.

Depending on our own goals and aspirations, we are all at different stages of that squiggly path. While some of us may already be at the finish line, others may just be taking their first step. The dilemma you might well find yourself experiencing is drawing comparisons to individuals who are at different stages of their journey. You then convince yourself they are better, more disciplined or have more willpower than you, rather than rationalizing that you're just *not quite there yet*. You look ahead at the finish line, at those clutching their gold medals, while you are just crossing the halfway point.

Often, comparisons might see you go against your better judgement or common sense. You ignore the fact that they started their journey a couple of hours, days, weeks, months, even years, before you embarked on your own. It might be that you have made a commitment to get fit ahead of the New Year. It's Day 1 of your running plan and you find yourself comparing yourself to Claire in the office, who has completed her second marathon. Maybe you have started out at a new workplace and draw comparisons between yourself and someone who has been in the job for two years. Or maybe you're a new mum, comparing yourself to a mum of three who just seems to have motherhood nailed.

Striving for imperfect perfection

Take a runner, for instance, who has recently completed the London marathon. Do you look back at their training schedule over the months leading up to the big day and rob them of that mammoth achievement based on those 'slow training runs' or 'the days they never made it out through injury'? No, of course not. Our journey does not, and should not, take away from the end result. That runner's purpose was to complete the London marathon, and while their journey getting there may have felt *less than perfect* at times, it offered them opportunity to learn, to grow and to complete it nonetheless.

An even simpler example: you buy yourself a bag. You put it down in a Tube carriage during a busy commute and it gets scuffed. Would you render the bag useless, chuck it away based on the fact that it has this scuff? No. While the scuff is far from ideal, the bag is still perfectly capable of carting your stuff from A to B and the scuff is accepted (albeit begrudgingly) as a blemish or flaw.

Setting yourself high standards

You wouldn't expect that never having run before, you would suddenly become capable of completing a marathon in record time. You need to prepare yourself for it to be a long learning process, during which you almost certainly will experience setbacks (getting a poor time, missing a run here and there and possibly sustaining an injury). Rather than enjoying the challenge of a journey, you might find you become fearful of making these 'mistakes', and, depending on how you interpret them, they may compound the idea that '*you are not perfect*' or that '*you are useless*' or that '*you can't ever achieve what you set out to do*'. This can damage your self-esteem, which sits on a knife edge between 'not making mistakes and being perfect' and 'making mistakes and not being perfect'. Your self-esteem suddenly relies on meeting these impossibly high standards that you set yourself.

Meet Nicola:

Nicola is 28, a nurse, a wife and a mum. She has recently returned to work after a period of maternity leave. Having to now navigate a career, a marriage and the responsibilities of being a mum, things are starting to take their toll. Nicola is constantly told 'I don't know how you do it' by her friends, family and work colleagues. She refuses to accept help because she perceives doing so as defeat – she should be able to manage it all. She worries about getting it wrong in all aspects of her life; what if work don't think I am as sharp as I once was, what if the nursery thinks I am selfish for packing my child off there, and what happens if my husband feels that I have lost 'it' (whatever 'it' was and attracted him to me in the first place).

Nicola finds herself constantly double-checking, if not triple-checking, anything she does at work. Procedures that used to take her no time at all now take twice if not three times as long, and that's if they even get completed at all, due to the fear of getting it wrong. She refuses to delegate, because she doesn't trust that others won't do it without mistakes and worries how this ultimately makes her look. She picks up her son from nursery and is straight into the kitchen to rustle up a home-cooked dinner. She refuses to prepare anything that has been in a packet because 'the perfect mum always makes stuff from scratch', which means it is all systems go as soon as she gets into the house. She can spend hours in an evening, browsing online stores to buy her son some clothes, worried about getting the wrong thing. Similarly, holiday bookings are always tricky. She finds that she is pawing over review after review to find the perfect holiday destination, for fear that the blame will be on her if they pick a rotten place to stay. Her husband jokes that it is lucky they even manage to book anything, with how long it takes her to decide on somewhere. The same goes for a simple family lunch out, and don't even get her started on a date night. It has created a rift between them both, with her husband often telling her to 'loosen up'.

I spoke to Nicola about the expectations she places on herself. She shared that she had 'always been the person that had it all and could do it all', and that she hadn't felt like that person since having her son. While she expected and accepted that her life would change after becoming a mum, she was worried how this would look to other people demanding of her time, particularly work. She feared that they might see it as her letting herself go, or allowing her standards to drop and not taking it as seriously. She felt this pressure at home and at work. She felt she ought to be able to do everything. While she accepted that she might need help (from her husband at home, and from work – by being more flexible about when she leaves), she equated needing help as not being trustworthy or competent. After all, in the past she could just be left to get on with things.

We reframed her 'asking for help and not being competent or trustworthy' as being conscious of her limitations, and surely that made her more trustworthy.

We conceded that Nicola was setting herself impossibly high standards, based on her previous roles (a wife and an employee), for fear that other people would perceive her as 'slacking' if she was seen to be dividing her attention even further. She gave each of her roles 100%, pushed herself to full capacity, and had very little room left to look after her own wellbeing. For Nicola, not aiming for perfection equated to her 'not trying' or 'not being bothered' – it was as black-and-white as that. There was no middle ground.

We reflected on what it might feel like for Nicola not to be perfect at all those things, not to always get it right, and not to be seen to be doing it all. While she initially found it difficult, Nicola was able to show herself more compassion. She was spinning a lot of plates. Her life had changed, but her benchmark hadn't. Nicola worked towards re-setting this benchmark, taking into consideration all her current responsibilities, which meant that she was no longer holding herself ransom to her pre-child, even her pre-married, self.

Ask yourself

Do you consider yourself to be a perfectionist?

....

....

....

Do you always think that you should give something 100% or you might as well not bother at all? Think about times when you have done this.

....

....

....

Do you spend a long time making decisions for fear of getting it wrong or making a mistake? Think about times when you have done this.

....

....

....

Do you find that even the simplest of tasks can take longer for you to complete than for someone else because you are constantly checking and changing things?
Think about times when you have done this.

....

....

....

Do you struggle when other people are tasked with making a decision, and find yourself trying to micromanage or influence it rather than sitting back? Think about times when you have done this.

....

....

....

After you have done something, do you find yourself being self-critical and thinking it's not good enough and you could have done better?

....

....

....

Do you find that you always put things off because you are worried it is not the right time?

....

....

....

If the situations described sound all too familiar, it may be worth considering whether the need to feel perfect is the source of any possible stress you may be experiencing. If so, then it may be an idea to think about how you ease the pressure you put on yourself to be perfect, and how you in turn embrace being imperfectly perfect.

Letting go of perfect

What is the worst thing that can happen from you not getting something right or doing something that is not 100% perfect?

This is not to say that you can't set yourself ambitious goals or uphold high standards, but it is about determining at what cost and being realistic about the journey that gets you there, i.e. that it won't come without its challenges.

Here are some tips for managing a more imperfectly perfect journey:

Expect and accept that you will make mistakes along the way. This is normal. Mistakes are an opportunity to learn and not a determinant of your self-esteem or self-worth.

Reframe how you view mistakes. Change your understanding of what it means to 'make a mistake'. Getting it wrong sometimes doesn't mean that you are useless, nor does it mean that you will never achieve what you set out to, rather it is a means of telling yourself that something is not quite right and instead it should be viewed as a tool for personal development, a way of learning for 'next time' rather than ruling out 'the next time' altogether.

Next time you find yourself comparing your imperfection to someone's 'perfection', **remind yourself of that path analogy** and that you are at different stages of that path. The path will look different for all of us. We will all feel challenged by different aspects of that journey; some of us may require more pit stops than others, but either way, as long as you embrace the obstacles that come your way, you will make it to the finishing line.

Start to enjoy the journey. Hopefully, if you have come to a place of accepting that there will be setbacks along the way, you will feel less apprehensive about those bumps in the path because you now come to expect them and embrace them.

THE 5 SENSE CHALLENGE:
when has perfectionism stood in your way?

Think about the last time you felt that you had *failed* at something, whether it was a personal, professional or social goal. Using the path below, highlight what you felt the setbacks on your journey were, and what, ultimately, if at all, led to you throwing in the towel and not achieving your goal. Think about what went well, the peaks. Why weren't the peaks strong enough to override the setbacks?

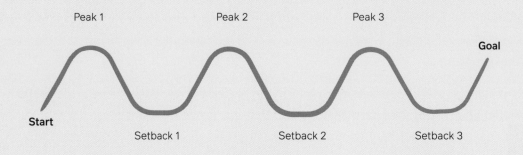

Looking back at your journey, do you think you may have given up too soon?

Do you think the standards you set yourself were realistic?

If you could go back and do it again, knowing what you know now, what would be different? *Could you pull that all-nighter to study for an exam, even if you spent half the night procrastinating anyway? Maybe you would have allowed yourself a more chilled evening or an early night, and not considered either of those as you 'taking your foot off the pedal'?*

'Unsuccessful' goal	Standards you set yourself	Did you meet those standards?	What did I do well?	What 'set-backs' meant that you threw in the towel?	Continuing to think about this unmet goal? What could you do differently?

Feel confident in your own skin

Do you believe confidence is something you either have or you don't? Do you ever look at someone and think, *'I wish I had their confidence . . .'* or *'I wish I didn't care what people think as much as I do.'*

If I were to pluck you from your current job and stick you into a new role with no word of warning, how would you feel? Or if I removed you from one friendship group into another? Chances are most of us would feel a little unsure about our new set-up. You may doubt your ability to carry out the new role or to find common ground with complete strangers, and may even wonder whether you would be any good at it. That's completely normal.

Someone who is naturally quite confident will *still* experience uncertainty or a bout of the *'what ifs'* when put in unfamiliar situations, the difference being that they believe that they can learn that skill (pick up that new job role or forge friendships) over time and eventually become proficient at it. Those who are less confident end up drowning in uncertainty and self-doubt, such that they don't have the belief that they can ever learn that new role or forge those connections. Their self-confidence becomes entangled in something that feels out of reach; it is based on their current skill set rather than having the self-belief or foresight that they could learn that new skill and might even be good at it in time.

Meet Lucy and Jack:

They are both temping at an office as administrators – manning the phones, typing letters, coordinating meetings and taking minutes. One morning, the team manager walks into the admin room and declares that she has been called out to another meeting across town tomorrow morning. She wants the team's usual meeting tomorrow to go ahead as planned, but needs someone to chair it. She wants Lucy and Jack to decide among themselves who that will be. She adds that 'this might happen a couple of times over the next month because the other team are really stretched'. 'I'm in my room if you want to check anything out beforehand', she calls out as she leaves.

Lucy and Jack stare at each other blankly. They are both feeling a bit uncertain, with having this dumped on them at the last minute. Neither are particularly sure whether they are 'experienced enough' to handle this new responsibility. Both worry about taking their boss up on her offer to 'check things out beforehand' – what if it highlights that I am no good at my job?

After a bit of a silent stand-off, Lucy suddenly offers to chair the meeting. She is not 100% sure but is willing to give it a go. She tells herself she can do it. Jack is relieved, to say the least.

Lucy jots down some questions that she has for her manager. They work together in sorting out a rough agenda for tomorrow that means that she isn't going into it blindly.

The morning of the meeting arrives and Lucy's nerves are awry. She pops to the toilet beforehand, looks herself in the eye head on, and tells herself: 'You will smash this.' She imagines the meeting going well, the pats on the back from her peers and the congratulatory handshake from her manager. She sits down, takes her place and the meeting starts. Jack looks onwards, taking minutes.

'Lucy seems so confident,' 'I wish I had the confidence to say yes,' 'I could never do anything like that,' he thinks.

Throughout the meeting, Lucy is second-guessing herself. She stumbles on a couple of the item agendas but manages to steer them through the meeting relatively unscathed. Lucy feels 'on top of the world', and motivated to take on the next meeting. Her boss commends her on a job well done the next day.

Both Lucy and Jack had the same starting point. They had the same experience, the same job and the same opportunity presented to them. They both felt uncertain – we've established that this is normal – but Lucy had the belief that while she didn't know everything there was to know at the beginning, she could begin to learn and develop those skills. She even fitted in some last-minute preparation with her manager, to help plan the meeting ahead of schedule. Lucy also accepted that despite making a few mistakes at the meeting, this did not define the meeting's outcome or its success. She was able to challenge this by reminding herself that she'd had little time to prepare. Lucy also engaged in some positive self-talk immediately before the meeting – 'You will smash this'. This gave Lucy the motivational push she needed to go in there and to do just that. Lucy being able to run that meeting relatively successfully, with little warning and preparation, will help spur her on to believe that she can do anything she sets her mind to; even if she doesn't have those skills to begin with, having the belief that she can learn them is all she needs.

Ask yourself

Think about a situation or time when you have felt under-confident. What barriers stood in your way?

....

....

....

What sorts of things ran through your mind as reasons why you couldn't do something or pull it off?

....

....

....

Knowing that it is your belief (rather than just your skills) that can stand in your way, would you do anything any differently?

....

....

....

THE 5 SENSE CHALLENGE:
recognizing our strengths

There is a common assumption that confidence is universal. If you are confident in one aspect of your life, surely you are confident in them all. You may feel confident toasting at your best friend's wedding in front of a roomful of guests, but *still* lack the confidence to speak publicly in a working capacity. It is important that in moments of self-doubt you are able to recognize the former (your strengths) and not discount them on the basis of a negative experience (or times where you have felt less than confident).

In the first column, write down your strengths. What are you good at? What are you capable of?

In the second column, write down what you would like to be able to achieve but are not quite able to yet. I have purposefully not referred to these as 'weaknesses' or 'failures'. By labelling these as weaknesses or failures it may render you powerless to change them. You might assume that because you are no good at them, you never will be, yet it is this willingness and belief in learning a new skill that is the key to our confidence in acquiring it.

Strengths	Would like to . . .

During moments of self-doubt or low confidence, return to this list and remind yourself of what you **can** do – what your strengths are – to put that self-doubt into context and to avoid you overgeneralizing that just because you struggled to speak out at that one team meeting, it doesn't mean that you will always struggle to do so.

The bathtub

Imagine you are sitting in a hypothetical bathtub surrounded by warm, soothing water. Each time you say something negative about yourself, the plug lifts a little and water spirals down the plughole. As you continue to talk negatively about yourself, more water drains away. You feel less comfortable (no longer surrounded by warm bathwater) and are more vulnerable (exposed and cold).

Imagine each time you positively self-talk, you are pushing that plug firmly down, so there is no chance of that lovely bath water escaping.

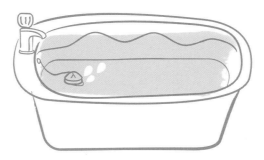

Think about what your own bath might look like. What negative thoughts stand in your way daily? How might you go about challenging these with your positive plug?

....

....

....

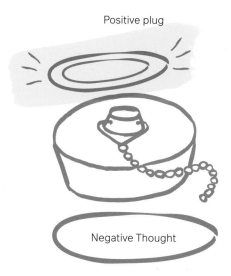

Positive plug

Negative Thought

While it might not be realistic to replace your negative self-talk with positive self-talk, you can determine how much importance you place on it. Remind yourself that your negative thoughts **do not determine your outcome** – *I can't do it* does not mean you can't do it. Acknowledge why you might be experiencing this negative self-talk and **be compassionate**. **Label what the negative self-talk is really trying to communicate**. Is negative self-talk before you meet your partner's friends really just fear of making a bad impression? Realizing this is the case will help weaken the hold that the thought has on you. **Plug your negative self-talk with a positive plug of self-talk.** Offer yourself a motivational phrase – *You can do it* – or think of a more specific instructional phrase that will help enhance how you act: *They'll love you* (motivational) and *talk to them about something you have in common* – your boyfriend – (instructional).

Lightening the load when feeling under pressure

Ever find yourself on a conveyor belt of should-dos and must-dos? What you do becomes constrained by rules you create for yourself that dictate your every waking move, and they can lock you into a cycle of guilt when you contemplate breaking them.

I know I fall foul of this myself. As a married working mum of one, I know that I have made life more difficult for myself than it needs to be. I feel that I must be the one that picks my daughter up from school, largely guided by the dreaded mum guilt. I believe that if I am not the one that picks her up, school will think I am a slack mum who prioritizes her work over her daughter. Even during busier periods at work, I still end up doing the drop-offs and pick-ups, despite the offer of help from family.

I struggle to accept help because accepting help would mean accepting that I don't have time for my daughter, and not having time for my daughter means that I am a bad mum. This means that I continue to overstretch myself and, come the end of the day, feel like a pressure cooker whose top may blow at any given moment.

I accept that I carry a lot of pressure on my shoulders – the responsibility of being the only one who drops her off and picks her up.

A particularly busy period at work forces me to address why I am not willing to accept support from eager family members. I convince myself that agreeing to the help would be letting her down – after all, I always drop her off and pick her up.

I can't seem to rationalize that accepting help on the odd occasion does not automatically mean that I am letting her down, nor does it mean that I'll have no time for her.

Even when I do pick her up, my work is often incomplete, which means that even when I am with her physically, mentally I'm not, with the laptop more often than not being fired up as soon as we get through the door.

I have forced myself to think about the situation more compassionately. I would almost certainly tell a friend in a similar situation to stop being so silly and accept the help. I know that I would probably be more disciplined about separating my work and home lives if I accepted help from family. It would mean that I could wrap up what I needed to at the office, so that when I did get home my attention on my daughter would be undivided.

I conceded that if I accepted the help from my mother-in-law to do the drop-off or pick-up even once a week, it would ease some of the pressure in my metaphorical pressure cooker. I even started to challenge my 'should-dos' and 'must-dos' with more compassionate explanations:

'My mother-in-law could help and enjoys being asked.'
Or
'I'm going through a busy patch at the moment, which means I need more help.'

I even removed the blinkers and was able to acknowledge that I had seen everyone from mums, dads, grandparents and nannies at the school gates picking up children. The rule that 'only mums should do the pick-ups otherwise they are bad mums' was one that I had created for myself and one that couldn't be translated to anyone and everyone. If I truly believed that I was a bad mum for not collecting my daughter, then by that reckoning, would every mum who did not collect their daughter from school be a bad mum? No, of course not. I realized that the only person being held to ransom by these high standards and expectations was me.

The pressure cooker

The pressure cooker will help you think about what unrealistic expectations you set yourself and the rules you live by that create pressure for you day to day. With nowhere for this pressure to go and no self-compassion or willingness to ask for help from others, this pressure continues to build, feeling increasingly overwhelming until your top or lid is blown. The exercise forces you to take the role of a compassionate friend and to think about what you can do to release some of that pressure you put yourself under and stop it spilling over and blowing that lid off.

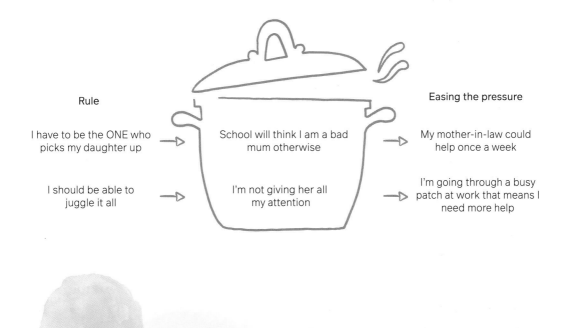

Rule

I have to be the ONE who picks my daughter up →

School will think I am a bad mum otherwise

Easing the pressure

My mother-in-law could help once a week →

I should be able to juggle it all →

I'm not giving her all my attention

I'm going through a busy patch at work that means I need more help →

Ask yourself

Have there been times when you have put yourself under pressure by setting yourself unrealistic rules and expectations – the should-dos and must-dos? Would you hold a friend or family member to these similar rules and expectations?

....

....

....

....

THE 5 SENSE CHALLENGE:
be kind to yourself

Write down a list of rules that you live by that leave you feeling under pressure. Start each of these with 'I should . . .', 'I must . . .', or 'I have to . . .' Jot these down on the left-hand side of the pressure cooker.

Write down why you stick by these rules. What is the fear that holds you to them, that stops you asking for help? Jot these down within the pressure cooker itself.

How might you ease some of that pressure on yourself? Play the role of a compassionate friend, and think about what advice you might offer a friend who found themselves in a similar situation. Jot these down to the right of the pressure cooker.

Every time you find yourself feeling under pressure, refer back to this pressure cooker. Think about the rule that is driving this pressure in, and not allowing it to escape, and play the role of the compassionate friend. What would you offer a friend in a similar position? Would you tell them to take a break? Would you offer to lend them a hand?

THE 5 SENSE CHALLENGE:
the art of delegation

As proven with the simplest of tasks, like a school drop-off or pick-up, I struggle with delegation. Feeling like you are the only one who can or ought to do something can be incredibly overwhelming. For me, I know it shows itself in me being snappier and feeling like I am letting people down. Learning to let go of something you feel you ought to be able to do yourself can be difficult, but more often than not it is the perfect antidote to mounting pressure.

Can you relate to the struggle of letting go and delegating? If so, the next time you find yourself feeling under pressure, ask yourself whether you are the *only* person who can do this task or whether there is someone else you can call on to help.

Create a to-do list at the start of each day, following the pattern on the exercise overleaf.

Record your wellbeing temperature where red is urgent, needs actioning today, blue being it would be nice to do, but not essential that I do.

Can you delegate tasks to anyone else?

Think about **who** can help you, with **what** and **how**? You might like to use the WWH method (see page 152) to help you with this.

I have identified my mother-in-law (**WHO**) to help me feel less overwhelmed with the pressure of needing to finish work before collecting my daughter (**WHAT**), by picking her up twice a week (**HOW**). This simple delegation means that my wellbeing temperature has gone from a RED to a much more manageable YELLOW.

Make sure you record your wellbeing temperature **after** you have put the support in place, to consider whether it is something worth continuing with, particularly if your wellbeing temperature comes down.

To-do	Before	Who can help?	Why this person?	What can they help with?	How can they help?	After

Stop feeling like an impostor

Ever experienced 'impostor syndrome' – moments where you doubt yourself and your abilities and fear that you're going to be *found out*, uncovered as a fraud for not knowing as much as you claim to, or not being as experienced as you claim to be? This might even be despite a wealth of skills, qualifications and achievements under your belt. It can be incredibly disabling, leave you feeling on edge, and get in the way of you being able to enjoy the exciting opportunities that come your way. You start to believe you are an impostor. You play your successes down, attributing them to sheer luck, discounting all the hard work that has gone in to achieving them.

Instead of focusing all your energy on why you shouldn't have been put forward for something, ask yourself 'Why not me?'

Meet Ellen:

Ellen has recently been promoted at work to senior makeup artist. She has landed her first major beauty campaign and is excited, if not a little nervous, about this. The first day on set she turns up and is surrounded by her junior glam squad, who are all poised to take directions from her on what look they should be going for. The models start to file in. Ellen freezes. Suddenly she is flooded with self-doubt. 'How am I here? Surely they made a mistake, I shouldn't be the one leading this campaign, there are plenty of other artists that are far more qualified than I am.'

I spoke to Ellen about her self-doubt and feeling like an impostor. She told me that she 'felt like a fraud', therefore she 'must be one'. This feeling utterly consumed the day for her. She feared that she would 'slip up', that she would miss the brief of the brand and that they would uncover her as the unqualified, inexperienced artist she was starting to believe she was.

Ellen agreed that she often took her feelings on as her identity. She labelled herself.

'I feel . . . therefore I am . . . '

'I feel like a fraud, therefore I am a fraud.'

We considered what feeling like a fraud had meant for her that day. She described not feeling able to celebrate a success that she knew would be an exciting opportunity for anyone. She felt that she was spending too much time on each of the models at the risk of delaying the shoot, for fear of getting it wrong. She didn't break for her lunch and instead found herself frantically searching makeup tutorials on YouTube, to perfect her technique ahead of the next model coming through the doors. Not at any point through all of that did Ellen congratulate herself on a job well done.

Ask yourself

Have there been times when you have felt like an impostor? What did it feel like and how did it make you act?

....

....

....

....

I spoke to Ellen about her self-doubt and feeling like an impostor. She told me that she 'felt like a fraud', therefore she 'must be one'.

THE 5 SENSE CHALLENGE:
why not me

If you frequently experience impostor syndrome, next time those feelings take charge give this 'why not . . . ' exercise a go.

This exercise helps challenge that inner voice of '*They've made a mistake, it can't be me*' and grounds a more powerful stance of '*Why not me?*' When you are put into a new situation, face a new challenge or your expertise is called upon, fear of failure or '*being found out*' can take over. This means that you rarely enjoy the success or commend yourself on a job well done.

Instead of focusing all your energy on why you shouldn't have been put forward for something, ask yourself '*Why not me?*'

Ellen was able to challenge her doubts with the following 'why nots . . .'

Fraud feelings	Why not me?
I don't know enough	I am an award-winning makeup artist
I'm going to slip up and then they will know I am not as good as they think I am	I have made mistakes along the way but have still been offered this opportunity
I'm not good enough	People have told me I do a great job, and I wouldn't have been asked to do this had I not been good enough
They are all looking at me like what does she know?	They are probably looking at me for guidance

I also encouraged Ellen to use a 'worry curfew' (see page 150) to stop those 'feeling like a fraud' worries in their tracks, to avoid the inevitable procrastination and ruminating that they would lead to, that would distract her from what it was she ought to be doing. We also focused on the importance of embracing imperfection and not equating this to not being capable or deserving of success.

Complete your own list of 'why nots' below and have these to hand to remind you of why you are deserving of successes that come your way. You may also find it helpful to put in place a worry curfew and worry dump, to avoid those feelings of being an impostor devouring time and energy at the expense of what else you have to be getting on with in the day. Be boundaried about when you can worry about feeling like an impostor and you will feel more in control of situations where self-doubt arises.

Fraud feelings	Why not me?

Chapter 5

TASTE

Food glorious food

We can't talk about taste without addressing a link between how we feel and what we eat. We have all experienced those pre-exam or job interview nerves that make our stomach turn at the thought of having anything to eat. For some of us the opposite is true – food becomes a source of comfort in testing times or the focal point of celebration in happier days.

I see patients daily who have struggled with their relationship with food for various reasons; from those whose increase or decrease in appetite may be down to their depression, to those who have developed disordered relationships with food, which in turn impacts their emotional health.

There is no question that the relationship between what we eat and our mental wellbeing is a complex one. To help navigate this tricky terrain I have invited sports and eating disorder specialist dietitian and author of *Orthorexia*, Renee McGregor, and Jenny Rosborough, registered nutritionist and head of nutrition at the Jamie Oliver Group, to share their expertise with us.

Do you think the types of food we eat can affect our mental wellbeing?
Jenny: Food affects our health and wellbeing in more than one way. Firstly, food gives us the energy we need to survive. A varied diet is the best way to ensure you're getting all the nutrients your brain and body needs to develop and function well. Some nutrients play a more specific role when it comes to how we feel. For example, carbohydrates are the body's preferred source of energy and also contain many important vitamins. Protein foods contain iron, and if we don't get enough our bodies become fatigued and we can feel lethargic. Fruit and vegetables contain a range of nutrients – aiming for a rainbow of colours is an easy way to ensure variety! And don't forget to stay hydrated. Dehydration can impact concentration and lead to tiredness, whereas high caffeine intake can impact sleep and in turn impact mood. The food we eat often also reflects our cultures, traditions and sense of belonging. This too is important for wellbeing. It is also true that how we feel can impact what we eat. Striving for a 'perfect' diet can be detrimental to overall health when, in reality, balance and variety, achieved by eating food which is

affordable and practical over time is key. This is all part of the bigger picture of other lifestyle factors like sleep and exercise. Remember that it is our overall dietary patterns and eating situations, not a specific food or 'magic bullet' nutrient, which impacts how we feel.

Is there such thing as the perfect diet?

Renee: So it's not as simple as eating in a specific way every day to ensure good health; it's also about responding to your internal cues, something many of us have lost sight of due to the abundance of external cues via social media. Our bodies are like an ecosystem, they are constantly changing, so we need to change with them as well as working with our environment. This means not stressing if while you are on holiday you drink a little too much or have dessert every night; it is one week in 52. So in reality the 'perfect' diet is about having a healthy attitude towards food and appreciating that what we eat in one moment is not going to impact us immediately.

How regularly should we be eating and what should make up the bulk of our plates?

Renee: In general our body requires food every 3–4 hours, in order to prevent blood sugar fluctuations but also to ensure optimal hormonal response. If you continually leave long gaps between eating, it can increase your stress hormone, which in turn can have a negative impact on the hormones which are necessary for so many functions within the body, such as immune, bone and cardiovascular health.

In general, the guidelines around food have not changed: our diets should be based around starchy carbohydrates; plenty of colour in the form of fruit and vegetables; protein sources such as fish, chicken, pulses, eggs and tofu, and red meat occasionally; good fats such as nuts and their oils, avocados, oily fish and seeds; dairy or soya alternatives for optimal bone health. And while foods containing sugar should be kept to a minimum, this means they should make up the smallest component of your nutritional intake; it does not mean that you should never include them.

For each meal, our plates should roughly consist of one third carbohydrate, one third protein and one third vegetables. This is a useful guide to bear in mind if you are eating out.

THE 5 SENSE CHALLENGE:
your weekly shopping list
(as advised by Jenny and Renee)

The information below is a guide based on the UK government's Eatwell Guide. It demonstrates the balance of different food groups required for the majority of the population – not necessarily at every meal, but across the course of a day or week.

The portion sizes provide a handy guide, but remember that individual needs differ. It's not necessary for the majority of the population to weigh or take a prescriptive approach to food.

Remember that your shopping list should include foods that you enjoy and that are feasible to prepare. Food does not have to be fresh or organic – food that is frozen or canned (in water) can be just as nutritious, prevents food waste and is easy to prepare on a busy day.

Have a look at the label on the front of the packet and look for green and amber labels for fat, saturated fat, sugar and salt. A healthy balanced diet can still include foods high in fat, sugar or salt, such as chocolate, crisps or cake – it's about how often and how much!

Think about what you eat over a typical week and jot it down on these pages.

Notes

....

....

....

....

Using coloured pencils, draw the corresponding food group symbol beside each item on the list as instructed in the following pages.

How diverse was your diet last week? Don't be disheartened if you don't tick off each of the food groups or recommended portion sizes opposite – this exercise is here to show you where improvements can be made.

Looking back at your list, what didn't you get enough of? With this in mind, write down a list for next week's shopping and make sure you tick off your requirements as on the previous page.

Did you eat any starchy carbohydrates?
Starchy carbohydrates include foods like potatoes, bread, rice, pasta, breakfast cereals, oats, couscous and noodles. Aim for 3–4 portions per day, and opt for wholegrain where possible for extra fibre!

A portion is:
- 2 handfuls of dried pasta shapes or rice
- A bunch of spaghetti the size of a £1 coin, measured using your finger and thumb
- The amount of cooked pasta or rice that would fit in two hands cupped together
- A baked potato about the size of your fist
- About 3 handfuls of breakfast cereal

Put a brown tick next to any sources of starchy carbohydrates you ate last week.

Did you eat a variety of colourful fruit and vegetables?
Use the list on page 190 to jog your memory. Variety is key – eat a rainbow of colours. We should be aiming for 5+ portions per day.

A portion is:
- Approx. what you can fit in one hand
- 150ml (a small glass) of juices and smoothies; if you do opt for a juice or a smoothie, these should not be used for more than one of your 5 a day.

Put a coloured dot next to each fruit and veg item on your list to see how many colours you ticked off last week.

● ● ● ○ ●

Did your diet include protein sources?

Protein foods include beans, lentils, chickpeas and other pulses, eggs, meat and fish, meat alternatives, plus nuts, seeds and hummus. Aim for 2–3 portions per day. Eat a variety of protein sources and aim for 2 portions of fish a week (allergies and food preferences aside), including one oily fish like salmon or mackerel.

A portion is:

- A piece of grilled chicken breast or salmon about half the size of your hand
- 2 boiled eggs
- 200g of baked beans

Put a black square next to any protein sources you ate last week.

■

Did you eat any dairy or alternatives?

Dairy foods include milk, cheese, yogurt, cream cheese, and dairy alternatives such as soya drinks, soya yogurts and other plant-based drinks such as almond milk. If you prefer plant-based dairy alternatives, look for those fortified with calcium and ideally other nutrients too. Aim for 2–3 portions per day.

A portion is:

- A piece of Cheddar cheese about the size of two thumbs together
- About 3 teaspoons of soft cheese

Put a white square next to any dairy (or dairy alternative) you ate last week.

☐

Did you eat any sources of good fats?

This might include: nuts, nut oils, seeds, avocado, oily fish.

Put a tear shape next to any sources of good fat you ate last week.

Portion sizes are based on the British Nutrition Foundation's 'Find your balance: get portion wise' guide. They're based on the requirements for an average healthy female adult. Visit www.nutrition.org.uk/healthyliving/find-your-balance/portionwise.html for more info.

Red

Apples ☐

Beetroot ☐

Cranberries ☐

Cherries ☐

Pomegranates ☐

Radishes ☐

Red cabbage ☐

Red grapes ☐

Red onions ☐

Red peppers ☐

Rhubarb ☐

Strawberries ☐

Tomatoes ☐

Watermelon ☐

Orange

Butternut squash ☐

Cantaloupe melon ☐

Carrots ☐

Grapefruit ☐

Mango ☐

Orange peppers ☐

Oranges ☐

Papaya ☐

Peaches ☐

Pumpkin ☐

Sweet potatoes ☐

Yellow

Bananas ☐

Honeydew melon ☐

Lemons ☐

Pineapple ☐

Sweetcorn ☐

Yellow peppers ☐

Green

Apples ☐

Asparagus ☐

Avocados ☐

Broccoli ☐

Cabbage ☐

Celery ☐

Courgettes ☐

Cucumbers ☐

Green beans ☐

Green grapes ☐

Green peppers ☐

Kale ☐

Kiwi ☐

Lettuce ☐

Pears ☐

Peas ☐

Rocket ☐

Spinach ☐

Blue

Aubergines ☐

Blackberries ☐

Blueberries ☐

Figs ☐

Plums ☐

Keeping it regular

We can all find ourselves caught short – where a balanced plate feels far from possible. Perhaps we've returned from holiday to an empty fridge? Or we rushed to a concert straight from work and are desperate to stave off hunger pangs but don't have a snack to hand? Maybe we are simply feeling too anxious to eat.

Now there may be times when you have legitimately overfilled yourself at the previous meal and just didn't feel hungry. Here I'm referring to the times when you have forgone a meal or snack and when you know you *ought* to have eaten something. You may even have experienced negative effects from not having done so, such as headaches, irritability, feeling light-headed and struggling to concentrate.

We have already touched upon the importance of eating regularly, not only to help with fluctuations in blood sugar, but also for optimal hormonal response. So, if you find that you are someone who routinely skips meals or snacks, that might be a good place to focus.

Ask yourself

How often did you skip a meal or snack in the last week? Why was this?

....

....

....

....

....

....

How did going without that meal make you feel or behave? *Record your wellbeing temperature.*

....

....

....

....

....

....

Are there patterns to when you skip? Perhaps every week there is always a meeting that overruns, or a midday flight or Friday night drinks with a friend that can see you waiting 6–8 hours between meals.

....

....

....

....

....

....

....

....

....

THE 5 SENSE CHALLENGE:
plan ahead

At the start of the working week, look at your diary for the week. Highlight in red where stopping to eat something might be difficult, bearing in mind that suggested 3–4 hour window between meals. Being aware of these hot spots means that you can prepare, ahead of time, and avoid being caught short.

- Prepare a meal at home to take with you if you know that access to shops, cafés and restaurants, or time to visit them, is limited.

- Where you envisage there will be long gaps between meals or long shift patterns, or if you'll be going to the gym straight from work, make sure you pack a snack in your bag to tide you over.

- If you are visiting a new area or travelling, spend some time researching the area and possible stop-offs online, and plan your meal and snack times around these.

Think about the difference this preparation, once you have put it in place, makes to your ability to focus and concentrate on subsequent tasks.

What impact does it have on your wellbeing temperature?

Throwing out the rule book

Eat meat. Don't eat meat.
Eat plant-based. Don't eat plant-based.
Fast. Don't fast.

There are so many mixed messages when it comes to what we should be eating that it is a wonder we manage to eat at all. When I look at my little girl, I am struck by her innate ability to honour her hunger and fullness cues. If she is hungry, she eats. If she is not, she will clamp her mouth shut. If she fancies something sweet, she roots around in the cupboards at home to find something that will satisfy her sweet tooth. If she doesn't fancy a pudding, she pushes her plate away, guilt-free.

We all started out like this, with the innate ability to listen to and honour our body's needs. Where did it all go wrong? For many, as we grow up, the messages relayed to us via the media and marketing all stand to distort our relationship with food.

We may develop rules around food, live in cycles of gorging and restriction, of guilt and unashamed joy; the euphoria of losing weight and then the pang of guilt when we break what were unrealistic rules or goals in the first place.

For many of the patients I see, food often falls into two separate camps; it is either good or bad, clean or a cheat, on plan or off plan. There is no in-between. They associate 'good' foods with how they make them feel or what they believe they will help them achieve, whether that is looking great or feeling better or just because it's cool.

Similarly, they associate 'bad' foods with ones that will derail them from those efforts to slim down, get fitter or be on trend. We apply moral labels to food. We're *'being good'* or *'are good'* if we eat foods that we perceive to be just that: good. And we are being *'naughty'* or *'bad'* if we eat something we perceive to be either of those things.

Why should what you eat be a determinant of your character? If I choose to eat a chocolate bar, am I a bad person? Why should we berate ourselves over *'lacking willpower'* or *'having no self-control'*, based on our desire to eat something?

Invariably creating such rigid, unrealistic rules around the food we eat can set us up to fail; it can create and sustain unhelpful and unhealthy relationships with food. When we perceive ourselves as bending the rules *that one time*, it can see us falling off the wagon:

'I might as well eat all the chocolate now because I've blown it.'
And
'I'll be back to "clean eating" tomorrow.'

That is until the next slip-up. It's that 'black-and-white' thinking that sets us on a difficult path of binging and restriction. Each 'slip-up' further compounds our 'poor' self-control, which can wreak havoc on our self-esteem. We admit defeat, throw in the towel, binge. We feel guilty, we berate our lack of self-control. We restrict. It becomes a vicious cycle.

'I have no willpower. I am useless.'

What makes this cycle even more difficult to break is the validation we get from those around us, well-intentioned family and friends who praise us for our self-control when we turn down the offer of dessert, or from those #bodygoals saved images on social media that remind us of why we set upon this path in the first place.

We may convince ourselves that we are actually eating what we fancy and believe our new lifestyle is 'not restrictive'. To the outside world, we are *'disciplined'*, *'have self-control'* and are *'good'*, but on the inside we are flapping and crumbling under the pressure of pretence. The decision we make to pass on that slab of chocolate cake when *'you really could have done with it'*, is the very decision that ends up tormenting us for the remainder of the day. How many of us have successfully passed on that chocolate cake only to scramble around later trying to find something that will equally satisfy the urge for a sweet hit that we denied ourselves earlier? Come the end of the day we end up succumbing to temptation, and the inevitable *'I've had something bad now. I've blown it, so I may as well keep going'* binge follows. Not long after, the guilt ensues and then the inevitable self-loathing, compounding our low self-esteem. We can feel utterly defeated over our *'lack of willpower and self-control'*.

Chances are you may read this and think, 'I am lucky that I have a very positive relationship with food.' If you do, I would still encourage you to give the next exercise, 'What do you fancy?', a go, as for some of us the restrictions around food may not be as clear-cut or as obvious on the surface.

Ask yourself

Clear your mind. Imagine you are coming round to mine for dinner. An impromptu decision. I haven't told you what we are going to have. We are going to have whatever I have in.

How do you feel? Record your wellbeing temperature.

....

....

....

....

What is your instant thought? Do you try to compensate for the unknown by restricting what you eat earlier in the day or dragging yourself to the gym?

....

....

....

....

I don't have an open-plan kitchen/living space, which means you will be oblivious to the cooking process. You won't know what I am going to make until it presents itself on a plate to you. You won't know how much fat I am going to use in the cooking process. Now, genuine allergies and intolerances aside, would you eat what I presented you with? What are the 'what ifs' going through your mind?

....

....

....

Record your wellbeing temperature.

Do any thoughts pass through your mind of what you need to 'do' when you get home to compensate, or are you able to accept this as 'just another meal'?

....

....

....

Some of you might be worrying, what if she just serves me a plate of carbs?
So what if I do?

....

....

....

What if she adds too much oil?

So what if I do?

....

....

What if there isn't enough protein?

So what if there isn't?

....

....

What happens if there isn't a single veg on the plate?

So what if there isn't?

....

....

Do your comments surprise you?

This simple exercise helps you to address your food biases and the rules and restrictions you may knowingly or unknowingly place on yourself. While we are only talking about one meal here, invariably these rules and restrictions may well impact you from the moment you wake up to the moment you go to sleep. It might even be the very thing that keeps you up all night worrying.

What living by these rules can mean

Food is crucial. It is fuel. Not only do you need it to function day to day, to optimize your physical health, but it also has massive implications for your mental wellbeing. Your own relationship with food can impact other areas of your life, including your family relationships, friendships and working and social lives. In the scenario played out in the previous pages, the fear, if you experienced it, of what would be presented to you may impact your spontaneity in going out for food with a boyfriend, grabbing a bite to eat with a work colleague or sharing a bag of popcorn at the cinema. This may create missed opportunities to wind down, work or socialize. You may repeatedly turn down social gatherings with friends and family due to the fear of eating out. You might disguise your difficulties well, scouring the menus beforehand, dictating where and when you eat to your friends. While on the surface it may appear that you are eating a broad range of foods and have a real flexibility in what you eat, you may be forced to make allowances elsewhere that others don't see; the restriction earlier in the day to '*allow you to eat normally later on*' or the hour of spin class the following morning to compensate.

In my experience of working with a broad range of patients, I have seen families and friendships torn apart over what is often one of the most complex relationships an individual will experience in their life, the one that they have with themselves, the food they eat and their body.

Ask yourself

To consider whether you might have a problematic relationship with food, ask yourself the following questions:

When you wake up in the morning, do you eat what you genuinely want or what you feel you ought to?

....

....

....

....

Do you find that after eating a meal you rarely feel satisfied and are already planning the next meal or snack?

....

....

....

....

Do you feel guilty for eating a certain food product or food group?

....

....

....

....

Do you find yourself labelling food as 'good' or 'bad'?

....

....

....

....

Do you find yourself calling out your choices to others? *'I'm trying to be good'* or *'I'm having a cheat or a naughty day'*?

....

....

....

....

Do you find that when you have ordered food you are staring longingly at what the other person has ordered and wishing you could have ordered that [insert desired food choice here].

....

....

....

....

Do you track your food intake and does this tracker ultimately decide whether you have permission to eat something or not?

....

....

....

....

Do you find yourself frantically scouring a food menu before a meal out, for anything other than curiosity, excitement or dietary intolerances or preferences? Can this often be a deal breaker as to whether you choose to go out or not?

....

....

....

....

Do you find yourself having to 'compensate' for eating certain foods? You might tell yourself that '*I can only eat x foods because I was naughty the night before*', or you might tell yourself that you have to work extra hard at the gym or go for a run to burn off what you ate.

....

....

....

....

THE 5 SENSE CHALLENGE:
the food thought tally

For the next 24 hours, record how many thoughts you have about food, even if it is just a fleeting thought, using the log below. How does this thought make you *feel* – tally your response under the appropriate coloured heading. If the thought made you feel miserable (e.g. *I wish I could have had that chocolate cake at lunch*), tally it as red, but if this thought made you feel positive (*I'm so excited about going out for food this evening*), tally it as blue or green.

The food thought log

					Total

Once your 24 hours are up, look back at your log.

Are your thoughts about food predominantly negative (red) or positive (blue)?

....

....

Do you think more or less often about food than you thought?

....

....

Ask yourself

Imagine that the brain below represents ALL your thoughts in a typical day. Shade the proportion that you feel is occupied by thoughts about food, where 100% is all day every day.

Is there room for you to think about anything else? What other thoughts occupy your mind – thoughts about your family, relationship or work? How much space do these occupy in comparison? Is thinking about food at the expense of these?

....

....

....

....

Next time you find yourself spending time thinking about food, stop the thought in its tracks and ask yourself what you really would like to be thinking about.

What parts of your brain do you wish you had more access to and spent more attention on?

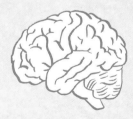

If your thoughts about food come at the expense of being able to do something with others, think about what positives they are potentially keeping you from. Allow yourself to remove food from the equation and remind yourself of what going for brunch with a partner, or having lunch with work colleagues, can also offer – having a laugh, social connections, better working relationships.

Where do these rules come from?

What are the specific thoughts that you have around food?

....

....

....

....

You may well find that there are common themes around the types of food you can or can't eat:

'I can't eat that because it is a carb and I am going on holiday next week.'
Or
'I can't eat cake because it has sugar in.'

You might have certain rules around when to consume food, depending on the place and time, or the company you are keeping.

'I couldn't possibly have a dessert because everyone will think I am greedy.'
Or
'I can only have that post-workout.'

Think back to your early relationship with food. How did you view food when you were younger? Did you have a carefree attitude to what you ate? Was there more flexibility and variety in your diet?

....

....

....

....

Are there any key moments that stand out for you that you can attribute your rules and relationships with food to? Comments from family, friends, teachers, work colleagues or complete strangers, growing up?

....

....

....

....

Use the timeline overleaf to pick out key memories. *Record your wellbeing temperature for each of these.* There may be key stand-out memories where you recall being able to enjoy your food (blue), if only briefly, for instance where your mood was already on a high and you were eating among family or good friends, like your wedding day; or there may be red memories, such as when a peer at school called you 'fat' as you were tucking into your chips at lunchtime as a teen.

Think about how this memory has shaped or changed how you view food, for worse or for better as you have got older.

Food thought timeline

Birth

Memory:
....

Wellbeing temperature

Thought/feeling/behaviour
....

....

Memory:
....

Wellbeing temperature

Thought/feeling/behaviour
....

....

Memory:
....

Wellbeing temperature

Thought/feeling/behaviour
....

....

Memory:
....

Wellbeing temperature

Thought/feeling/behaviour
....

Present
....

Meet Tess:

Tess describes feeling stressed (RED) every time she comes in from work. Without so much as a second thought, she roots around her snack drawer and devours anything and everything she can get her hands on. She tells herself that she 'shouldn't really eat that' (biscuits) because they are 'bad', but then convinces herself that she has had a tough day and therefore deserves to. Eating the forbidden biscuit makes her feel good initially. It tastes good and allows her to temporarily forget about the stresses of the day. That is, until the guilt sets in and the self-loathing begins. 'I have been naughty. I have no willpower. That's it, I've blown it. I may as well eat shit for the rest of the day then.' This then triggers the inevitable binge where she gorges past the point of feeling comfortably full. Cue more of the self-loathing and the inevitable restriction the following day.

Tess recalls that as a child whenever she had a bad day at school she would rush through the door, often in tears, be encouraged to have a 'treat', and would sit devouring said treat while her mum reassured her that everything would be OK. And by and large her mum was always right. Tess would return the next day and any of the previous day's trivial disagreements with friends would be forgotten. Tess lost her mother in her early 20s, and while she had moved out of the family home and kitchen-counter conversations were no longer possible, she still found comfort in being able to pick up the phone to relay or rant about her experiences of the day.

We spoke about Tess's interpretation that her 'reaching for food was a marker of her lack of self-control'. Tess was able to accept that the binge-and-restrict rollercoaster that she had found herself on, not long after her mum's death, wasn't just about the food and had very little to do with a 'lack of willpower or self-control' – there were lots of difficulties at play that manifested or showed themselves in her behaviour around food.

We conceded that in moments of stress, talking with her mum, often over a packet of biscuits, was the tonic Tess needed to bring her stress levels from a raging RED to a buoyant BLUE. Tess had not yet come to terms with her mum's death, so in moments of stress she found herself desperate for the instant reassurance that these experiences (sitting at the kitchen counter, eating biscuits or picking up the phone) gave her, the biscuits in particular holding some childhood nostalgia.

If that wasn't difficult enough, Tess had also been conditioned to view these foods as 'bad' through societal and marketing messages, such that she had restricted them for most of her teens and early adulthood. Every time she succumbed to temptation and 'broke the rule', i.e. had one biscuit, a full-blown binge would follow. She would feel guilty at having done so and this would simply compound how low she was feeling.

'I still feel stressed, and I feel even worse and worthless now that I have devoured a whole packet of biscuits.'

Tess added that she 'wasn't even hungry', and found herself berating herself while feeling physically uncomfortable. This would then ultimately leave her feeling more stressed than she had to begin with.

For Tess, the solution didn't lie in the usual 'how to' articles in glossy magazines, such as 'how to control your cravings' (that never worked anyway), but rather in her trying to decipher what she was seeking out instead. It was also important for her to come to terms with how labelling her foods as 'good' or 'bad' meant that when she did reach for 'bad' foods in moments when she craved nurture and nostalgia, she interpreted this as 'having no self-control', compounding her already flailing self-esteem. This rendered her unable to show herself the self-compassion she deserved in those moments – 'I've had a tough day', 'I miss my mum at moments like this, she always knew what to say to me.'

By opening Tess up to this, she was able to accept that she needed to think about how detrimental her labelling of foods was to her. Over time, she started to rationalize that no food was inherently good or bad for her. It had been marketing and media messages that had drilled this into her from a young age. She started to challenge her black-and-white thinking around food, which weakened the moral value she placed on it. She would have one biscuit but challenged that 'it was one biscuit', that 'it wasn't bad and neither was she' for having it. This meant that she didn't set about a path of self-destruction by eating the entire packet purely because she may as well now that she had been 'bad'.

Tess was also able to re-evaluate how she responded to stress. She came to realize that what she was really craving were those nurturing conversations with her mum. While eating biscuits was an act of nostalgia and gave her a temporary lift, actually it was short-lived because she hadn't truly satisfied her true hunger (an unmet emotional need). We mind-mapped who Tess might be able to offload to after a tough day, and she was able to identify three close friends who might be able to lend a listening ear, over a packet of biscuits of course. This meant that the next time Tess returned from work feeling stressed, instead of holding on to all of this until she got home, she was able to reach out to a friend and offload. She could make plans to see them straight away and found herself feeling considerably less stressed and calmer having spoken to them, so that by the time she got home the urge to binge felt less pressing.

Spotting your food labels

Have you ever fallen into the labelling trap? Do you find yourself either having '*all of something*', or cutting it out completely only to spend prolonged periods of time pining for it? When you did eventually succumb to the '*forbidden fruit*', was this in response to a true physical hunger – stomach rumbling, feeling light-headed – or was it in response to an emotional hunger, to suppress feelings of stress or feeling tormented, so that all you could think about was the said food item?

When I was in my 20s I enlisted the help of a personal trainer. I had lost my way in the gym a little and needed some workout inspiration. Unbeknown to me, part of the PT package involved looking at my diet. I wrote down my week of food as requested and presented it to him at the following session.

'You eat an awful lot of fruit, don't you?'

'Is that bad?' I asked him.

'Yes – fruit is just pure sugar.'

He started to write with his red pen and suggested some changes that I could make. The new 'plan' included no fruit. I remember returning home to my husband announcing that we had done the 'whole eating thing' wrong. The fruit bowl disappeared overnight, and for a good couple of years after I avoided what I was led to believe were the 'wrong' or 'bad' foods in favour of what the trainer perceived were 'good' (and pretty tasteless) substitutes.

This very conversation had a profound impact on how I ate and shopped. I feared fruit – something that I had grown up to enjoy. I felt guilty when I 'caved in'.

The turning point for me came when I fell pregnant. A lot of the substitutes I had been encouraged to use were not suitable during pregnancy, and something just clicked for me – why had something as natural as fruit been deemed forbidden? I was flummoxed to find I didn't really have an explanation other than that this was what I had been told. Knowing how impressionable and vulnerable children can be, I didn't want my daughter to see me demonize fruit and not provide a rational explanation as to why we never brought it into the house and why she wasn't encouraged to eat it. Crucially, I didn't want to be responsible for her labelling foods and assigning moral value to food.

Have you ever beaten yourself up over '*being bad*' or given yourself a pat on the back for being '*good*' and resisting temptation? What external factors hold you accountable to these rules?

Food is crucial. It is fuel. Not only do you need it to function day to day, to optimize your physical health, but it also has massive implications for your mental wellbeing.

THE 5 SENSE CHALLENGE:
freeing yourself

Our labelling of foods can be reinforced by subliminal or conscious messages around us that validate our reasons for eating or not eating certain foods. This can be anything from conversations with friends who revel in the 'let's treat ourselves' or 'let's be naughty' after a tough day, to the latest social media post demonizing a particular food. The more messages we have to this effect, the stronger and more ingrained our belief can become and the more difficult it can be to shake off. The solution? Start to cut these messages off at the source and free yourself from the trap of being held accountable to them.

Unsubscribe from emails and mailing lists related to diet culture. Stop parting with your money in the name of the latest fad and what it promises. If you need a reminder of how to do this with confidence, refer back to Chapter 3, SMELL: Smelling the bullshit (page 120).

Curate your social media feed. Is your feed representative of all body types? Do food pictures and diet plans occupy your feed and highlights reel? Does your highlights reel tell you anything about you as an individual? Are you defined only by the food you eat? Ensure that your social media platforms reflect all facets of your life.

Stop assigning a moral value to the food you eat. Challenge your own rules as and when they crop up. When you find yourself standing in front of that deli, longing for a pasty but settling for a salad instead because you are trying to be 'good', call yourself out: '*This food cannot determine what I am like as an individual.*'

What would a friend or family member say? Do body stats feature on our CVs? The food we eat has almost become an extension of our identity, but how many of your family or friends, if asked to recount your personal qualities, would describe your food intake, what you look like or how much you weigh as your defining feature? '*She's really lovely, really good at her job. She eats clean and is really ripped.*'

Similarly, if you are applying for a job, how many prospective employers wish to hear that you 'avoid carbs' and will make a judgement of you based on that? Do your dietary choices have a bearing on how able you are to do your job? If other people don't see the food you eat as an extension of your identity, why do you?

Get rid of those objects that tell you what and how much you can eat. Are you:

- **A slave to apps?** Delete food-tracking apps that hold you accountable for every bite.

- **A slave to a diet plan**? Has this plan been devised for anyone and everyone? Who has created this for you? Have you even met them? Is it based on a common assumption that 'everyone wants to be beach body ready' or that 'everyone wants to shift the Christmas bulge'?

- **A slave to your kitchen scales**? Limit your use of kitchen scales to only the absolutely essential, to execute a recipe rather than as a tool to limit your portion size.

- **A slave to your bathroom scales**? Does the number on the scales determine what and how much you can eat for the rest of the day? If so, get rid.

- **A slave to your wardrobe**? How many of us are triggered to restrict what we are eating based on how the clothes in our wardrobes fit? Wear clothes that fit, and get rid of those that hold us to account and serve as a reminder of what we ought to be doing. '*I don't fit in to these any more therefore I haven't been good.*'

Challenge why you give these objects so much power. They reduce the whole you to a number. Your bathroom and kitchen scales, if you use them, don't know the first thing there is to know about you as an individual – all those strengths you know to be true about yourself are suddenly negated by a number. It doesn't matter if you are thoughtful, hardworking or loving – for as long as you weigh x pounds less, that's all that matters, right? Sounds ridiculous when you put it like that, doesn't it?

You might find it difficult to unsubscribe from these all at once.

You might prefer to take a more graded approach and build yourself up to ditching them completely. Refer back to Chapter 3, SMELL: 'Sweet Smell of Success' (page 126) for strategies on how you might do this.

The drug and supplement trap

Alcohol

A higher proportion of us are choosing to adopt a teetotal lifestyle. The UK's Office of National Statistics reported that since 2005, the proportion of Brits between the ages of 16 and 44 adopting a teetotal lifestyle has increased, with 20% of us claiming to be teetotal in 2017 (a staggering 10 million). While it is difficult to identify a reason for this growth in teetotalism, it has been postulated that an increased awareness of the harmful effects of alcohol, changes in licensing rules and a spark of wellbeing and wellness trends, particularly on social media, may have a role to play.

Many of my patients describe drinking as enhancing how they feel. When they are happy and in the company of good friends, drink lifts their mood. It can make them feel relaxed and more confident in new situations. However, when they are low, drinking sees their mood spiral even lower.

Alcohol is a depressant, and for some it can exacerbate feelings of stress and anxiety. Alcohol can affect how you think, feel and subsequently act. It may also lead to some of us developing more chronic difficulties with low mood and anxiety.

When you think about alcohol, how do you feel? Record your wellbeing temperature.

If you drink, do you like to drink? Would you class yourself as only a social drinker or do you drink most days? Do you sometimes find yourself being coerced into drinking when you really would rather not?

Meet Penny:

Penny has not long started a job in the City. She hasn't been much of a drinker since her university days, but in among client lunches and after-work drinks she has found herself drinking more regularly. While it has certainly helped Penny feel more confident, particularly when meeting new people, the effects of drinking every day are starting to catch up with her. She is finding her sleep to be quite unsettled. She is waking up in the morning still feeling quite groggy, and doesn't feel as 'on it' at work the following day. She feels sluggish, and she swears she feels more anxious. Penny doesn't always feel she is able to say 'no' to a drink. She is not addicted, but rather there is the pressure from others that she ought to be drinking. Rather than face the awkwardness of being asked why she is not drinking, Penny just perseveres, accepting drinks when offered regardless of how it makes her feel.

I spoke to Penny about her drinking and she told me she would rather go without it.

Penny shared her fear that by not drinking she will be perceived as less committed to her job (entertaining clients), or as a bore. She concluded that no one had told her as much but this was the assumption she had drawn herself.

We spoke about where Penny's beliefs around not drinking stemmed from. Penny told me that whenever she didn't want to drink at university she would be called a 'bore' or a 'spoilsport'. She also found that she wasn't particularly sociable unless she had a drink inside her. Penny believed that in order to appear fun to other people, and to ensure that the conversation didn't run dry, she needed to drink. She shared that there had been occasions when she had met up with friends during the day and didn't have very much to say to them. This only served to compound this idea that she was only interesting when she had a drink inside her.

We reflected on Penny's experiences and conceded that these friendships weren't friendships in the true sense of the word and were built around a perceived shared interest, namely drinking. They could laugh at things that were not funny, dare each other to down shots and dance like no one was watching, but fundamentally the similarities ended there. The reason that Penny did not get on with these people in the cold light of day was not because she was a bore for not drinking, but rather because the alcohol masked pre-existing flaws in the friendships.

Penny's experience highlights a couple of points, namely that we can take on completely different identities when we have had a drink inside us, which can sometimes be the identity preferred by others. This may exacerbate insecurities we have about ourselves in situations where the common interest (the drink) is removed. It also introduces this idea that drink can often be about meeting someone else's needs rather than our own – we ignore our gut instinct (that tells us not to drink). We end up harbouring resentment towards the person who has weakened our resolve, as well as feeling disappointed in ourselves for not having the confidence to stick to our guns, and that's even before the hangover has had a chance to creep in.

Ask yourself

Do you drink? Do you notice that the effects vary depending on the company you keep and whether you do or don't want to drink?

....

....

....

If you find yourself routinely giving in to peer pressure to drink, what are the barriers that get in the way of you sticking to your guns?

....

....

....

Why someone might be coercing you to drink

Often other people's insistence on you drinking is more than likely down to their own biases. They may believe that *you can't possibly go on a night out unless you have had a drink*. Perhaps they have come to expect certain desirable behaviours from you when you drink and assume that these won't be there if you choose to remain sober – '*if you don't drink then you won't be able to do drunk karaoke*'. It might be that your decision to remain sober causes them to feel insecure about how being the only one drinking may appear to you or others; a fear of judgement. By trying to successfully coerce you into having '*just one drink*', they may feel more relaxed that they have the green light to do so rather than being forced to consider whether they also ought to be steering clear of alcohol given your own decision to do that.

If they are not drinking, should I not be either?

If they are worried about the negative effects that drinking has on them, should I be too?

This can be a difficult reality to face up to, particularly because the suggestion to not drink has not inherently come from them, but has been called into question indirectly and implied through you deciding not to.

THE 5 SENSE CHALLENGE:
to drink or not to drink – learning to respectfully decline

Ever find yourself bowing to the pressures of drinking when you would rather not? Ever predict the effects on your mood when you choose to cave in? Do you *just know* you will feel anxious for the remainder of the night or that you will be paying for it the following day?

Next time you are faced with the option to drink and you are in two minds as to whether to do so, allow yourself to take a temporary pause. Ask yourself:

Why am I drinking?

....

....

....

Am I drinking for myself?

....

....

....

Or to appease someone else?

....

....

....

....

How will drinking in this particular situation make me feel? Record your wellbeing temperature.

Remember, appeasing someone else and simply being happy that you have made them happy or got them off your back does not constitute you 'drinking for yourself'.

If you are not drinking **for yourself**, think about what the potential consequences of doing so might be – will it make you feel low rather than giddy? Will it make getting up early with the kids more difficult?

....

....

....

....

Handling 'that' conversation

An easy way to avoid the inevitable 'are you having a drink' question may be **dodging that social invite altogether**, when you foresee that there might be an expectation to drink.

Whether it is meeting a good friend, a work function or a party, stand by your decision not to drink and hold in mind that this is a decision that **you have made** for yourself. You shouldn't be coerced into changing that to placate someone else.

Consider whether the pressure to drink is **explicit** or **implied**. Is someone pushing a shot glass into your hand and asking you to '*down it*' (explicit), or is the pressure based on your own assumption that others will be drawn to the fact that you are not and take issue with it (implied)?

Be firm with your decision if someone encourages you to drink or if they press for reasons why you are not. **Don't feel you have to come up with a million and one excuses to justify your decision**, as this might suggest to others that you are *fumbling around for excuses* and have a resolve that could be weakened. If the request to drink is repeated, be polite, repeat back what you have told them and do not feel pressurized to waver.

If you feel uncomfortable in the situation, then you are well within your rights to leave, regardless of your relationship with the other individual. There is no circumstance where drinking is deemed absolutely essential. We all have the right to make our own decisions and for these to be honoured and respected by those around us. You should not feel coerced into doing a complete 180 on something that you know through your own experience is likely to make you feel worse.

Caffeine

Caffeine is often hailed as the world's most used (and abused) drug. It is a stimulant drug that most of us (myself included!) use daily to help keep us alert, enhance our performance and combat fatigue. It is available not only in teas and coffees but can also be found in energy drinks, colas, chocolates, protein supplements and energy gels. Even so-called decaffeinated alternatives to teas and coffees still contain small amounts of caffeine, with the caffeine dose in one cup of decaf up to 30% the dose of a regular cup.

Second to screens, caffeine is the next common culprit I contend with when speaking to my patients about their difficulty getting to sleep. The sleep process is initiated by our loss of daylight as well as a pressure to sleep created by a build-up of a chemical called adenosine in our brain. Adenosine binds to micro-sites (or receptors) in the brain, creating that indisputable urge to sleep. Caffeine, however, works by blocking adenosine from binding to these receptors. This means that adenosine continues to build up in your brain but has nowhere to go. That is, until the caffeine has worked its way out of your system, when the receptors once again become available and are saturated by the accumulating adenosine. You are then overcome with an insurmountable fatigue and need to sleep, aka the caffeine crash or come-down.

I know personally that I have to strike a balance with caffeine – one cup over my usual 2–3 cups of tea/coffee a day can find me feeling jittery and struggling to sleep. On the other hand, one of my sisters is quite content with an after-dinner espresso that seemingly has little impact on her sleep.

I invited Renee once again to share her expertise.

What are your thoughts on caffeine? Should we avoid or limit it?
Renee: This very much depends on the individual and whether you are a responder or non-responder; some of us metabolize caffeine more readily than others. It can take up to 7 hours for just half the caffeine in your late-night coffee to work its way out of your system. This explains why a late-night coffee for some can spell disaster and keep us wide awake, and for others has very little impact. If you are the former, you'd be wise to have your last coffee no later than early/mid-afternoon if you are aiming for a 10 p.m. bedtime.

Caffeine is often used to enhance performance. We know it takes 40 minutes for levels to peak, so you would do well to time your caffeine consumption 40 minutes prior to when you require performance to be optimal. In sport, the optimal dose is around 3mg/kg of bodyweight.

Anecdotally I see a lot of people in clinic who find that caffeine makes them anxious. Is there evidence to suggest that caffeine has this effect?

Renee: Caffeine can cause palpitations in some individuals. There is good evidence that above 6mg/kg bodyweight, caffeine will have a negative impact on everyone. One of the big concerns is the increase in the use of energy drinks, particularly by teenagers, as these can have quite high doses of caffeine, combined with sugar, which can lead to fluctuations in blood sugars and to heart palpitations, which can mimic and exacerbate physical symptoms of anxiety.

Second to screens, caffeine is the next common culprit I contend with when speaking to my patients about their difficulty getting to sleep.

THE 5 SENSE CHALLENGE:
curb the caffeine

How regular is your hit of caffeine?

....

....

....

....

Do you have a cut-off time for your last drink?

....

....

....

....

If you find that you are an afternoon/evening caffeine drinker, think about how drinking makes you feel before, during and after. *Record your wellbeing temperature.*

....

....

....

....

To consider how frequent your caffeine consumption is and to help determine why you might find yourself reaching for that caffeinated beverage at a specific time, fill in the caffeine log below. Think about why you are having a drink. Is it to make you more alert ahead of a work meeting? To give you a boost after a poor night's sleep? A coffee date with a friend? Or perhaps you simply like the taste?

....

....

....

....

Record your wellbeing temperature before and after having a drink. Does that coffee before a stressful team meeting (RED) allow you to become more focused (BLUE)? Does that after-dinner espresso with friends (BLUE) suddenly see you bouncing off the walls come bedtime (ORANGE)? How do you respond to caffeine?

....

....

....

....

Time	Situation	Type of Caffeine	Why	Before	After	Thoughts

If you find that your temperature is consistently red or orange post-caffeine consumption, or you find yourself reaching for a caffeinated drink through habit, procrastination or boredom, try to substitute it with a decaffeinated alternative. Be mindful that some decaffeinated teas and coffees, however, may still contain caffeine.

Is it worth considering whether your late-night caffeinated beverage is really a sign that you should call it a night and get some sleep instead? What alternative activities might prove a better option for you? Look back at your evening curfew (page 144) to think about non-stimulating activities that you can do instead.

....

....

....

....

Supplements

The role diet has to play in optimizing our mental and physical wellbeing is often marketed as going beyond the food we eat, with the mention of supplements never far from earshot. Figures in the last four years suggest that the UK's vitamin and supplementation market is worth more than £450 million and growing, with almost two-thirds of us taking some form of supplement daily or occasionally each year. As someone who finds the supplementation arena a difficult place to navigate, I invite Renee and Jenny once again to share their expertise.

Is there a role for prebiotics and probiotics in enhancing cognitive function and improving our mental wellbeing?

Renee: I think we are not yet able to extrapolate the data of the studies we do have; these are predominantly mice studies. Prebiotics are often overlooked but are necessary for probiotics to work. There is lots of evidence around both prebiotic and probiotic use in improving gut microbiome and this is having a positive impact on digestion, inflammatory bowel disease and immune health in athletes, but with regard to brain function it is still early days; it looks promising but there are no human studies currently. There is a definite link between the gut and the brain (gut-brain axis) but we need more research. That being said, there is no harm in taking pre- and probiotics as there are no long-term negative consequences.

Is there a role for supplementation?

Jenny: Apart from vitamin D, which everyone should supplement with during the winter months, we can generally get all the nutrients we need from a balanced and varied diet. However, there are some specific population groups who will need to supplement. For example, those following a vegetarian or vegan diet will need to supplement the nutrients which are predominantly found, or which are more available, in meat and fish, such as omega 3 (essential fatty acids), iron, calcium, vitamin B12 and iodine. Check with a health professional to find out more about supplements you may need.

Revenge tastes so sweet

Can anger ever be a good thing?

Anger often gets a bad rap. A lot of the patients I see describe a great deal of shame if and when they experience anger. They perceive anger as a purely negative emotion, one that indicates that they have no resolve, no patience, or have lost control. While anger certainly has the capability to be perceived as negative (and potentially destructive) by ourselves and those around us, this is largely determined by how we respond to it. Before we consider what anger is really trying to communicate to us or to others in any given situation, let's consider the different ways individuals may express it.

The bottlers

If you are a bottler, you tend to stew or deliberate on your anger. You feel hurt by what someone has done and need some time to process what has happened. If you are a bottler, you tend to go quiet. You might reply that you are fine when probed, but feel far from it. You may find a quiet corner and deliberate over what you want to do. You might take days, weeks, months, in some cases years to try to make sense of how you feel. This might have an impact on your mood and how you then go on to act. As a bottler you might end up hurting yourself in the process.

The exploders

If you are an exploder, you will let it be known from the off how you feel. You might shout at the person or situation that has wronged you. You may be explicit in your anger and tell the person that you 'hate them' or that 'they've done this' to you. You might get verbally and physically aggressive. You may throw objects and your behaviour might be quite destructive. As an exploder your behaviour can often become the focus of the situation and mean the original situation that led to the anger (being lied to by a friend or family member, or not getting that promotion) can get forgotten about and is replaced by your 'unreasonable behaviour and response' instead.

The relievers

As a reliever you might try to find a way of channelling your anger or reducing it. You may choose to work off your anger in the gym or go for a walk. You might turn to less helpful coping strategies, such as smoking or drinking, that you feel will help 'settle your nerves' or 'take the edge off', but it is easy to see how these sorts of strategies might be misused and be seen as the only way to manage difficult emotions.

While anger certainly has the capability to be perceived as negative (and potentially destructive) by ourselves and those around us, this is largely determined by how we respond to it.

Ask yourself

Have you ever felt angry? What does anger look like for you? Do you consider anger to be a positive or negative emotion?

....

....

....

....

Think about **why** you get angry.

Is it a way of expressing frustration at yourself?

Is it a way of letting someone know that they have upset or hurt you?

Is it a way of eliciting power and control over those around you?

Or do you find yourself irrationally and helplessly displacing your anger on to innocent bystanders through frustration that you can't direct it at the person who has actually caused you pain?

....

....

....

....

How does your anger show itself? Are you a bottler, an exploder or a reliever?

....

....

....

How does experiencing anger **leave you feeling**?

Does getting angry make you feel like you've lost control?

Do you feel guilty for hurting someone as a result of your anger?

Do you resent the person or the situation that has made you feel angry?

....

....

....

Think about a situation where you have experienced anger, where you feel crossed by someone or something. This can be as simple as someone swiping your seat on the Tube.

Record your wellbeing temperature. How did you respond? Did you bottle, explode or relieve?

....

....

....

What did you hope for from the situation?

....

....

....

'By getting angry, I hoped that . . .'

What was the reality?

....

....

....

Did the person apologize? Did they get angry or defensive? Did it escalate into a slanging match?

....

....

....

Do you think the outcome would have been different if you had responded differently? If you had explained why you felt hurt rather than exploded, would it have led to that individual being apologetic rather than defensive?

....

....

....

Directing our anger at others

Anger is a normal human emotion but can often be a response to another underlying emotion or feeling; the 'what's really going on?' When someone has hurt you or you feel hard done by, you might find yourself going over what they have done in your mind, ruminating. It can often be the only thing that you think about.

Why have they not apologized?

Do they think things are OK between us?

They'll get their comeuppance.

You might even wind yourself up in anticipation of the apology that you expect. I know that when I have become irritated with my husband for leaving a pile of dirty plates in the kitchen sink, I feel like my silent treatment (I'm a bottler) should just be picked up on by him. I might drop hints left, right and centre that only serve to wind me up even further when they fall on deaf ears. I might end up resenting him, ignoring him, being passive-aggressive and internalizing my anger. What I fail to realize is that through this, through my own anger largely and not relaying this to him, I stand to hurt only myself in the process. Whereas communicating why I am angry ('why can't you just wash your dirty plates rather than leaving them in the sink for me to do?') and working towards a solution ('can you either just wash them or put them in the dishwasher?'), I avoid the bottling that can see my anger come out in less than desirable ways, and doesn't impact our relationship in the way that being irritable and passive-aggressive might.

THE 5 SENSE CHALLENGE:
giving yourself permission

If you find yourself caught up in a cycle of vengeance, address this two-fold by considering **how am I hurting** (the emotive side) and **what do I want to do about it** (the practical side – the goal).

Label it: what's really going on

My irritability towards my husband stems from frustration and feeling like I am taken for granted. Uncomfortable as it may be to label what's really going on and to admit that it is frustration that is fuelling the anger, it allows my husband to empathize with my situation rather than just seeing and having to contend with my rage. Similarly, anger from not being picked to be bridesmaid for an upcoming friend's nuptials stems from hurt and disappointment; it is important that these emotions are given the opportunity to come to the forefront and are not masked by the 'anger'.

Does this person know about it?

Communicate with the person who has hurt you. Don't expect them to mind-read. By getting it out into the open, you offload how you feel, avoid harbouring resentment and give them opportunity to rectify the situation or redeem themselves.

Why has what this person done upset you? Was it that you didn't expect it from that particular individual? Has it made you look silly? Have they shattered the trust between you? Does it go against the values you hold important in a friend, family member, partner or work colleague? Does it remind you of someone who has hurt you in the past?

It is important to be really clear about why this action by this particular person has made you feel the way that you do. By being clear in your own mind as to why you feel this way, it can make communicating this to the perpetrator of your anger easier and help with moving forward more positively, should that be what you wish.

THE 5 SENSE CHALLENGE:
learning to move forward

Draw up a list

Once you have been able to establish why someone's actions have made you feel a certain way, **think about what continuing to punish them is achieving.** Jot down the pros and cons.

Situation	Pros to remaining angry	Cons to remaining angry

Stop getting personal

Tit-for-tat and name-calling. We've all been there. A disagreement turns personal and before we know it we are five names deep into a slagging match. Continuing to hurl abuse at someone who has upset you will likely just get their back up; anger breeds anger. Instead of calling out the perpetrator on what they have said – '*You're an idiot*', '*You didn't deserve the promotion*' – try to practise communicating how it has affected you personally, as this will help them empathize with your situation and how they have contributed to that, rather than just feeling attacked.

'*You've made me feel like a mug.*'

'*I feel like I tried really hard for that promotion.*'

Forgive or forget

The next question may feel a little trickier to answer for some of you, but give it a go. **Do you want to forgive them**? Would you like to get to a place where you are able to move past this? Holding this in mind will allow you to keep in check more destructive anger and remind you to keep the lines of honest communication open.

Think about how things would change if you allowed yourself to accept what has happened. If you didn't shout, scream or give them the silent treatment, might it be easier to move on from this?

Turning the situation around

Can some good come from your anger? Have your feelings of anger shown that you were more interested in that job promotion than you gave yourself credit for? Perhaps a love interest kissing someone else has put things into perspective and made you realize you do want to be with them. Can you use the anger as a motivator to go hell-bent for that promotion next time it rolls around, or to ask that person out on a date, for instance?

Chapter 6

THE 5 SENSES PLAN: BRINGING IT ALL TOGETHER

Commit to it

Studies have shown that it can take 66 days (about 10 weeks) for a behaviour to become a habit (i.e. something that we do automatically without thinking) if we practise it daily. While this might seem like a mammoth task and it's all too easy or tempting to throw in the towel, it is important to remember that these difficulties didn't come overnight and are unlikely to disappear overnight either. What it will take is you chipping away at them over time, building your confidence by practising them daily so that they become habitual. Commit to these goals daily for the next couple of months. Patience and consistency are key, and the rewards will come.

Setting goals

Think about what goals you want to set yourself over the next 10 weeks. Look back at each of the senses and think about what difficulty you would like to focus on. *Where did you routinely find your wellbeing temperature in the red or orange?*

For each of these difficulties, what are the accompanying sense challenges that you can practise daily over the next 10 weeks? Jot these down using your 5 sense goal sheet (page 243).

Be specific about your goals

Ensure that the goals you set yourself are specific. While it is admirable and certainly ambitious to simply want to be more confident or to listen to your internal 'no' more often, these goals are too vague and don't allow you to put them into practice specifically and then objectively measure them. You want to be able, at the end of the plan, to see how far you have come, how far you have progressed, and to measure this easily. So instead you might adapt *'I want to learn to listen to my internal "no"'* to *'I want to learn to say "no" when I am at work and am asked to do something on the spot when I don't have my diary to hand'*. This specific goal is what you need to input into your goal sheet.

Beside each goal, there is space to jot down the accompanying two challenges that are attached to the relevant sub-sense. This is an example of how you might complete the goal sheet for 'listening to your internal "no"':

HEAR goal:	HEAR challenge 1:
I want to listen to my internal 'no' when I am asked to do something at work on the spot	generate an important list
	HEAR challenge 2:
	develop a 'no' checklist

Goal sheet example:

It is important to realize that while some of the difficulties we have uncovered within this book may not be a problem for you right now, you may well come across these at some point in your lifetime; there may be a time when you are feeling less motivated, feeling more affected by what you see on your socials, or may find yourself in an overly critical relationship, for instance. As and when these do crop up, you can dip in to the relevant sense chapters, read up about these in a little more detail and adapt your plan accordingly.

I recommend you set yourself no more than 5 goals in the first instance. Remember, you will be reviewing your progress regularly, so as and when difficulties are no longer problematic for you and become automatic (habit), you can choose new areas to focus on instead.

You might choose to focus on one sense.

You might choose to focus on one area from each of the 5 senses.

You might choose to focus on only one challenge for the full 10 weeks.

There is no right or wrong way to do the plan; it can be as bespoke as you want it to be.

You want to be able, at the end of the plan, to see how far you have come, how far you have progressed, and to measure this easily.

Goal sheet

| SEE goal: | SEE challenge 1: |
| | SEE challenge 2: |

| HEAR goal: | HEAR challenge 1: |
| | HEAR challenge 2: |

| SMELL goal: | SMELL challenge 1: |
| | SMELL challenge 2: |

| FEEL goal: | FEEL challenge 1: |
| | FEEL challenge 2: |

| TASTE goal: | TASTE challenge 1: |
| | TASTE challenge 2: |

Plan, plan, plan

Think about when a realistic time might be to sit down to plan and set out your goals for the next couple of months. Is it a Sunday evening? Perhaps a Friday evening after work?

Ensure it is at a time when it is unlikely to be trumped by other activities.

Set a reminder on your phone. Do it now. This is a meeting with yourself that is non-negotiable. In much the same way that you would commit to a work meeting, a medical appointment or seeing a friend, the same rules apply.

I will sit down on [insert date] at [insert time] at [insert location] to plan and set out my 5 senses plan.

Getting started: setting a 5-sense agenda for the day and taking your temperature

Each day: morning

Look at your goals each day.

Stick them down where you can see them, read them as soon as you get out of bed, over your morning coffee or on your commute, and think about how you might be challenged that day to put them into practice. Record your wellbeing temperature at the start of the day for each goal, in anticipation of the obstacles to come. Jot down any thoughts you have within your notes section.

	Daily notes	
SEE goal:		
HEAR goal:		
SMELL goal:		
FEEL goal:		
TASTE goal:		

Each day: evening

At the end of each day, reflect on how things have gone. Look back at your goal sheet. Have you been challenged by any of them? If so, how did it go? Has there been any progress (cooling of temperatures from this morning) or setbacks (rise in temperatures)? Perhaps we made a hasty decision that forced us back several steps. Rather than just be frustrated that this has happened and either move on straight away or swear profusely and give up, it is crucial that we are able to take a step back and reflect, i.e. think critically:

'OK, that wasn't great but why did that happen?' 'Could it have been prevented?' 'What could I do differently tomorrow or the following week that would mean I would avoid this?'

These are the sorts of things that you want to capture in your notes section, to allow yourself to set action points for the following day. It also enables you to celebrate those small wins that can often get forgotten about when we are only focused on just reaching that end goal.

Each week: reviewing your progress

Using the weekly review sheet below, shade in your wellbeing temperature for each of the days and for each goal set. This allows you to have a quick visual indicator of any cooling or warming of temperatures and a quick weekly snapshot of the progress you make over the coming weeks. Week 1 may be a sea of reds and oranges, and by week 8 you may be seeing more greens and yellows crop up.

Weekly review sheet:

SEE goal: 👁	Morning 🌡	Evening 🌡	Notes
	M	M	
	T	T	
	W	W	
	T	T	
	F	F	
	S	S	
	S	S	

HEAR goal:	Morning	Evening	Notes
	M	M	
	T	T	
	W	W	
	T	T	
	F	F	
	S	S	
	S	S	

SMELL goal:	Morning	Evening	Notes
	M	M	
	T	T	
	W	W	
	T	T	
	F	F	
	S	S	
	S	S	

FEEL goal:	Morning	Evening	Notes
	M	M	
	T	T	
	W	W	
	T	T	
	F	F	
	S	S	
	S	S	

TASTE goal:	Morning	Evening	Notes
	M	M	
	T	T	
	W	W	
	T	T	
	F	F	
	S	S	
	S	S	

When you review your progress from one week to the next, think about what you may need to 'practise' or work on the subsequent week. The questions you might ask yourself include:

- What went well this week?
- What challenges have I faced?
- How can I feel better prepared for these next week?
- What would I like to do more of next week?
- Have there been any measurable changes in any particular sense?
- Have I managed to bring down my overall temperature?

By the end of the plan you will have collated 10 weekly review sheets. Place them side by side.

- How have you got on?
- Have you managed to overcome any of the obstacles and reach your goals?
- If you haven't, have you at least managed to make some progress in the right direction? Remember, even if the progress is marginal, it is to be celebrated.
- If you haven't made the progress that you had hoped for in some of the areas, why was this?
- Did you set the bar too high? Have you placed unrealistic standards on what you hope to achieve? Have you made your goals specific enough?
- Have you been consistent in practising your goals daily?

Epilogue

LET YOUR SENSES BE YOUR GUIDE

The aim of the 5 senses plan is to leave you feeling more empowered to make proactive changes to improve your mental wellbeing, and to spot when and why you might be struggling. I hope that some of the skills you have developed within your bespoke plan will now become second nature and will leave you feeling more positive about yourself.

Because our mental health runs in peaks and troughs across our lifetime, you may come back to this book from time to time, whenever you are faced with a challenge or obstacle. The 5 senses plan is available to you in the good times and the bad.

For some of you, the information provided in this book won't be enough and some of the challenges you are facing may feel too great, even with the support of a loved one, family, friends and work colleagues. If you are struggling with your mental health, do not hesitate to seek advice from a professional (a doctor or a therapist), who will be able to assess you and guide you to the most appropriate support.

I truly believe that each and every one of us has the ability to live, and is deserving of living, a mentally healthier and happier life. The most important relationship we have in life is the one we have with ourselves. Look after that one and everything else will fall into place.

Be self-compassionate.
Embrace change.
Be patient.
Be consistent.
And let your senses be your guide.

REFERENCES

Chapter 1: See

Armitage, C., 'Evidence that self-affirmation reduces body dissatisfaction by basing self-esteem on domains other than body weight and shape', *Journal of Child Psychology and Psychiatry*, Vol. 53, Issue 1, January 2012, 81–8

Barger, S., et al., 'Social relationship correlates of major depressive disorder and depressive symptoms in Switzerland: nationally representative cross sectional study', *BMC Public Health*, vol. 14, 2014, article number: 273

Barnett, P. A., and Gotlib, I. H., 'Psychosocial functioning and depression: distinguishing among antecedents, concomitants, and consequences', *Psychological Bulletin*, 1988, 104: 97–126

Cao, H., et al., 'Screen time, physical activity and mental health among urban adolescents in China', *Preventive Medicine*, Vol. 53, Issues 4–5, October–November 2011, 316–20

Dove Global Beauty and Confidence Report, https://www.unilever.com/Images/global-beauty-confidence-report-infographic_tcm244-501412_en.pdf

'How heavy use of social media is linked to mental illness', *Economist*, https://www.economist.com/graphic-detail/2018/05/18/how-heavy-use-of-social-media-is-linked-to-mental-illness

Khouja, J., et al., 'Is screen time associated with anxiety or depression in young people? Results from a UK birth cohort', *BMC Public Health*, Vol. 19, 2019, article number: 82

Maras, D., et al., 'Screen time is associated with depression and anxiety in Canadian youth', *Preventive Medicine*, Vol. 73, April 2015, 133–8

Mental Health Foundation/YouGov body image report, https://www.mentalhealth.org.uk/publications/body-image-report/exec-summary

'#Statusofmind. Social media and young people's mental health and wellbeing', Royal Society for Public Health, https://www.rsph.org.uk/uploads/assets/uploaded/d125b27c-0b62-41c5-a2c0155a8887cd01.pdf

Stiglic, N., 'Effects of screentime on the health and wellbeing of children and adolescents; a systematic review', *BMJ Open*, Vol. 9, Issue 1

Teo, A. R., Choi, H., and Valenstein, M., 'Social relationships and depression: ten-year follow-up from a nationally representative study', 2013, *PLoS ONE* 8(4): e62396. https://doi.org/10.1371/journal.pone.0062396

Thomée, S., et al., 'Prevalence of perceived stress, symptoms of depression and sleep disturbances in relation to information and communication technology (ICT) use among young adults – an explorative prospective study', *Computers in Human Behavior*, Vol. 23, Issue 3, May 2007, 1300–1321

Vogel, R., 'Social comparison, social media and self-esteem', *Psychology of Popular Media Culture*, American Psychiatry Association, Vol. 3, 2014, No. 4, 206–22

Walker, M., *Why We Sleep: The new science of sleep and dreams*, Penguin, 2017

Zheng, F., et al., 'Association between mobile phone use and inattention in 7102 Chinese adolescents: a population-based cross-sectional study', *BMC Public Health*, Vol. 14, 2014, article number: 1022

Chapter 2: Hear

Hoffman, S. G., et al., 'The effect of mindfulness-based therapy on anxiety and depression: a meta-analytic review', *Journal of Consulting and Clinical Psychology*, 78(2), 2010, 169–83

Hoge, E., et al., 'Randomized controlled trial of mindfulness meditation for generalized anxiety disorder: effects on anxiety and stress reactivity', *Journal of Clinical Psychiatry*, 74(8), August 2013, 786–92

Chapter 3: Smell

Chang, A., et al., 'Evening use of light-emitting eReaders negatively affects sleep, circadian timing, and next-morning alertness', *Proceedings of the National Academy of Sciences of the United States of America*, 112 (4), 27 January 2015, 1232–7; first published 22 December 2014

www.headspace.com

Kredlow, M. A., et al., 'The effects of physical activity on sleep: a meta-analytic review', *Journal of Behavioral Medicine*, Vol. 38, Issue 3, June 2015, 427–49

Pretty, J. and Barton, J., 'What is the best dose of nature and green exercise for improving mental health? A multi-study analysis', *Environmental Science and Technology*, 44(10), March 2010, 3947–55

Stahl, B., and Goldstein, E., *A Mindfulness-Based Stress Reduction Workbook*, New Harbinger Publications, Workbook edition, 1 March 2010

Stubbs, B., et al., 'An examination of the anxiolytic effects of exercise for people with anxiety and stress-related disorders: A meta-analysis', *Psychiatry Research*, January 2017

Chapter 4: Feel

Hatzigeorgiadis, A., et al., 'Self-talk and sports performance: a meta-analysis', *Perspectives on Psychological Science*, June 2011

Matthews, G., Dominican's Department of Psychology in the School of Arts, Humanities and Social Sciences, http://energycut.com.au/business/wp-content/uploads/2015/02/Dominican-Research-Cited-In-Forbes-Article.pdf

Pham, L., and Taylor, S., 'From thought to action: effects of process versus outcome-based mental simulations on performance', *Personality and Social Psychology Bulletin*, first published 1 February 1999

Shi, X., et al., 'The relationship of self-talk frequency to communication apprehension and public speaking anxiety', *Personality and Individual Differences*, Vol. 75, March 2015, 125–9

Chapter 5: Taste

British Nutrition Foundation, 'Find your balance – get portion wise!' https://www.nutrition.org.uk/healthyliving/find-your-balance/portionwise.html

Health Food Manufacturers Association (HFMA). https://www.hfma.co.uk/media-events/industry-facts/

NHS Eatwell Guide, https://www.nhs.uk/live-well/eat-well/the-eatwell-guide/

Office for National Statistics, Adult drinking habits in Great Britain: 2017

Chapter 6: The 5 Senses Plan

Gardner, B., et al., 'Making health habitual: the psychology of "habit-formation" and general practice', *British Journal of General Practice*, 62(605), December 2012, 664–6

Lally, P., et al., 'How are habits formed: modelling habit formation in the real world', *European Journal of Social Psychology*, Vol. 40, 2009, issue 6

Walker, M., *Why We Sleep: The new science of sleep and dreams*, Penguin, 2017

ACKNOWLEDGEMENTS

My husband, Ravi – your unwavering love and support throughout this whole process has been immeasurable. For the last 12 years you have tirelessly championed me. From the arduous years of junior doctor training, the long slog of studying for membership exams and finally to celebrating with me when I secured my consultant job. You have been pivotal in helping this 'side hustle' of debunking mental health myths and public education come to life. From challenging me on Boxing Day 2016 to 'set up an Instagram platform and to stop bending your ear off about it', to liking and commenting on my posts, retweeting me and telling everyone who will listen what I am up to. You selflessly pressed pause on our box-set binge evenings even though it pained you, brought me vats of tea and nipped out to buy me chocolate to fuel many a late-night writing session. You have ridden the highs and lows, endured the tears (of which there were many) and the laughter and incurred my writer's block wrath. You have helped bring this book to life and provided me with some valuable material for it (!), and I could not be more grateful to you.

My daughter, Amelie – I love you so very much. You have enriched my life in ways that I could not even have imagined. I feel so incredibly lucky to watch you grow up to be the smartest, most loving little girl. You have supported me in more ways than you realize. From your unconditional love, your constant cuddles and kisses, and your witty chat, to helping make bedtime a breeze so I 'can do some work' and knowing 'not to touch Mummy's computer' – though your 6 a.m. get-ups still leave a lot to be desired!

My mum, Soheir, and dad, Sami – thank you for shaping me into the woman I am today. You have taught me so many valuable life lessons, instilled in me the importance of education and selflessly loved and supported me through the long, demanding (and costly) years of training. I love you both.

My sisters, Lena and Nadia – my loudest cheerleaders. Thank you for your constant love and support and for keeping me entertained with hours of daily WhatsApp chat and the sharing of childhood anecdotes. I love you both so very much.

My brother, Ibby – thank you for your love and support.

My mother- and father-in-law, Harjit and Surinder – thank you for enabling me to take on more opportunities than I could dream of by stepping in, often at short notice, to help with childcare and just telling me to 'have fun and not to worry'.

My brother-in-law Roop – thank you for all your enthusiasm, your social media shares and for being Ravi's 'translator' when he hasn't quite grasped the importance of certain opportunities that have come my way.

My brothers-in-law Jules and Charlie – thank you for your enthusiasm and support and for letting me rabbit on when Nadia and Lena have lost interest, having heard it all before!

My oldest and dearest friends, Lizi and Jess – you have given me so much love and joy over the last 16 years. You have been by my side for every major milestone – exams, graduation, first jobs, marriage, becoming mums – and I could not be more grateful for having you both in my life.

Renee and Jenny – your support in informing the Taste chapter has been so crucial in ensuring that the information I share is reliable, responsible and evidence-based.

My secretary, Lisa – thank you for organizing my life and making sure my day job runs swimmingly. I couldn't function without you!

Every colleague and every patient that I have had the privilege of working with – each one of you has inspired every fibre of this book.

To all my social media followers and anyone who has read an article, turned up to an event, downloaded a podcast, tuned in to the radio to hear me speak, thank you. Without your support and this platform, none of this would have been possible.

To the whole team at Penguin Life, who have believed in me from day one, shared my enthusiasm for this project and helped bring it to life. I will forever be indebted to you all for your support and am so very excited about the journey ahead.